Friction, Lubrication, and Wear of Artificial Joints

IMechE Tribology Group

Tribology is a term coined in 1966, and is briefly described as the 'Science and technology of interacting surfaces in relative motion and the practices relating thereto'. This very broad scope embraces the processes of friction, lubrication, and wear in all mechanical contact situations.

Tribologists are concerned with optimum machine design and maintenance leading to improvement in service life, safety, and reliability. A successful tribological approach is critical to the economics and operational reliability of industrial manufacture and processing. Indeed, an inadequate tribological approach on the part of designers, operators, or management can lead to unnecessary cost and other waste, machine and system failure, sometimes catastrophic, and the loss of life.

The Tribology Group of the Institution of Mechanical Engineers is of particular significance by virtue of its 'horizontal' nature and its consequent relevance across industries. This broad relevance is underlined by the circumstances of the Group's origin, when in 1971 the UK Department of Trade and Industry passed to the IMechE the promotion, awareness creation, stimulation of research, and international relations for tribology in the UK.

The Tribology Group Committee meets four times annually to conduct formal business but specifically to monitor progress and achievement in specific actions, propose current and future modifications to planning, introduce new initiatives, and identify emerging subjects of importance.

IMechE Medical Engineering Division

Health care is one of the world's biggest industries. The main aims of the Medical Engineering Division of the Institution of Mechanical Engineers are:

- to raise the profile of Medical Engineering and the Health Care industry both nationally and on an international front;
- to provide a focus for technology transfer, the exchange of information and ideas, and the dissemination of best engineering practice in the field of Medical Engineering;
- to promote Medical Engineering both within and as a career in itself, and the continuing professional development of engineers working in the Medical Engineering arena.

The IMechE Medical Engineering Division works closely with other institutions under the umbrella of AIME – the Association of Institutions concerned with Medical Engineering –which was created to co-ordinate the activity of its members and to provide a single focus for the medical profession in the UK.

AIME's role is:

- to promote technology transfer and industrial competitiveness in Medical Engineering;
- to promote research, development, and manufacturing in Medical Engineering;
- to work alongside the Royal Academy of Engineering UK Focus Group for biomedical engineering.

Working in conjunction with IMechE's Medical Division, the IMechE Tribology Group has organized seminars exploring new directions in tribology with potential applications for medical engineering.

More information on the work of the Tribology Group and the Medical Engineering Division can be obtained by writing to:

The Institution of Mechanical Engineers
1 Birdcage Walk
London SW1H 9JJ

Friction, Lubrication, and Wear of Artificial Joints

Edited by

Ian M Hutchings

Professional Engineering Publishing

Published by Professional Engineering Publishing,
Bury St Edmunds and London, UK.

First Published 2003

ISBN 1 86058 363 6

A CIP catalogue record for this book is available from the British Library.

MIX
Paper from responsible sources
FSC® C013604

Contents

Editor's Preface

The subject of this volume is one with which many of us are likely to be personally concerned. Every year more than one million patients worldwide have a joint prosthesis implanted, the majority of which are hips and knees. Within the UK alone, some 40 000 hips and 18 000 knees are replaced annually. These figures are likely to increase substantially as advances in all aspects of medical science lead to an increased quality of life, with demands for greater mobility, for more members of an ageing population. The tribology of artificial joints poses particular challenges to engineers, medical scientists, and clinicians, and it is clear that the subject still has considerable scope for further development. I hope that the contents of this book will provide a useful resource for those working in this important field.

The chapters published here result from papers presented at a meeting held at the University of Leeds in November 2000. I am very grateful to all the authors for agreeing to contribute to this book, to Dr Todd Stewart, who played a major role in organizing the meeting, for providing a Foreword, and to the staff of Professional Engineering Publishing for their efforts in bringing the book to press.

Ian Hutchings
GKN Professor of Manufacturing Engineering
Department of Engineering, University of Cambridge

Foreword

The meeting on 'Friction, Lubrication, and Wear of Artificial Joints – tribology meets medical engineering' was organized by the University of Leeds Institute of Medical and Biological Engineering and supported by the Institution of Mechanical Engineers. The concept of the meeting was to encourage cross-fertilization of ideas between conventional engineering and tribology, and biological tribology and biomedical engineering, with the common goal of increasing the longevity of total joint replacements. The one-day meeting had three sessions chaired by Professor John Fisher and was attended by an audience of approximately 90 researchers, industrialists, and clinicians from Europe and North America.

A plenary lecture by Dr Ian Hutchings provided a perspective on bio-tribology and an historical review. The first session began with Dr Joanne Tipper describing how particulate debris generated by the articulation of artificial joints elicits a biological response. The following three speakers, Dr John Williams (wear modelling), Dr Christian Kaddick (hip simulator studies), and Professor Gordon Blunn (knee simulator studies) provided an excellent background to the current status and challenges in implant tribology.

The second session concentrated on the use of alternative bearings and 'new directions in tribology'. Dr Simon Smith and Gerard Insley reported the wear of metal-on-metal and ceramic-on-ceramic bearings. Dr Susan Scholes spoke on friction of hard-on-hard and soft layer joints. Dr Zhongmin Jin discussed modelling of lubrication in prosthetic devices. The final session entitled 'Recent advances and novel tribological solutions for orthopaedic implants' began with Dr Peter Hatto and Andrew Jones speaking on the use of wear-resistant ceramic coatings in orthopaedics. This was followed by Robert Scott and Dr Claude Rieker who reported new methods for the measurement of wear in knee prostheses.

The plenary lecture and first session set the stage for the day, stressing the importance of devices which produce both low wear volumes and wear debris with a reduced biological response. The following two sessions focused on recent advances in the field. With conventional polyethylene bearings it was shown that surface finish and design can affect the lubrication regime to reduce wear. This is also true for metal-on-metal and ceramic-on-ceramic bearings. Under the variable tribological conditions of daily life, joint replacements may operate with fluid film, mixed, and boundary lubrication. With current technology the production of wear debris, therefore, cannot be avoided though it can be reduced. Experimental testing of prostheses is moving towards more physiological test protocols with multidirectional motion and micro-separation, producing laboratory results which are closer to clinical retrievals. Surface engineered coatings have had only limited success in the past, but current research has improved this technology significantly. Overall the meeting was very successful, with the subtitle '*tribology meets medical engineering*' justly chosen.

The meeting organizers would like to thank Alison Payton and the Tribology group from the Institution of Mechanical Engineers for their support and promotion of this publication.

Dr Todd Stewart
Senior Teaching and Research Fellow
Institute of Medical and Biological Engineering, The University of Leeds

1

Biotribology – A Personal View

I M Hutchings

Abstract

Biotribology includes all aspects of the tribology of biological systems. Articulating joints form vital components of many creatures, and similar types of joints are found in very diverse organisms. The aspect of biotribology of particular concern in this volume is its application to prosthetic human joints, of which the hip joint has received the most attention. This challenging field of engineering is still developing, and there will continue to be important contributions to it from the medical sciences, as well as from more conventional tribology.

1.1 Introduction

It is surprising that the word 'biotribology' or 'bio-tribology' does not yet appear in the dictionary **(1)**, although it was first used by Dowson and Wright **(2)** as early as 1973 to describe 'all aspects of tribology related to biological systems'. This definition is wide enough to encompass the tribology of natural joints as well as prosthetic devices of all kinds. In this introductory chapter we will take a very broad view of the subject, surveying the range of articulating joints found in nature before focusing on some aspects of prosthetic joints, in particular the hip joint, for human applications.

1.2 Articulating joints in nature

Articulating joints are important not only in animal locomotion, but also in motion at the cellular level. One of the most remarkable examples of a natural joint is in the motor illustrated in Fig. 1.1 which is found in some bacteria such as *Escherichia coli* and *Salmonella typhimurium*. These organisms are typically around 1 μm in size, and propel themselves by the rotation of long, helical flagella. They are the only biological structures known that use continuous rotation for the purpose of locomotion. The rotational speeds of the flagella, of which each cell may have up to ten, can be as high as 300 Hz, while the diameter of the motor that drives each flagellum is only some 45 nm. A great deal is known about the structures of these motors, which derive their energy from a flow of ions down an electrochemical gradient, but much less is clear about the tribology of the 'bearings' which allow free rotation at such small scales **(3, 4, 5)**.

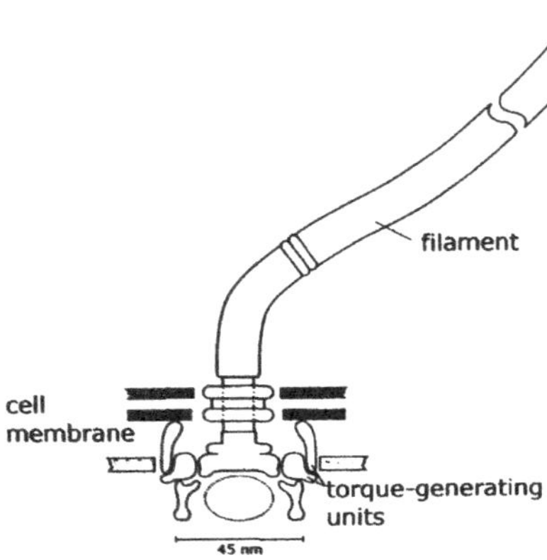

Fig. 1.1 The bacterial flagellar motor (after ref. 3)

In larger organisms free rotational motion is absent*, but there is remarkable consistency among the solutions to articulation which have evolved; the ball-and-socket joint, or at least an approximation to it, is very widely seen in nature. Arthropods and vertebrates have well-developed joints and the former, with exoskeletons predominantly of calcite, can form flexible linkages through rings of thin, flexible cuticle. Joints of this type can transmit only small forces, however, and in order to achieve a stronger articulation which can support the loads exerted in locomotion and in other activities such as feeding and defence, peg-and-socket joints have developed which have smooth cuticular bearing surfaces exposed to the ambient environment. Good examples of these are seen in crabs and lobsters, as illustrated in Fig. 1.2 **(6)**. An example of another invertebrate joint in a marine environment, of the ball-and-socket form which is closely similar to the synovial joint so common in vertebrates, is that at the base of the spine of a sea-urchin, which is used for both locomotion and defence, and shown in Fig. 1.3 **(7)**.

---

* Mythical creatures have no such limitations. The yale, first described by Pliny the Elder as 'the size of a hippopotamus with the tail of an elephant and the jaws of a boar' and later widely seen in medieval heraldry, possessed swivelling horns with a rotational mobility greater than any known animal joints.

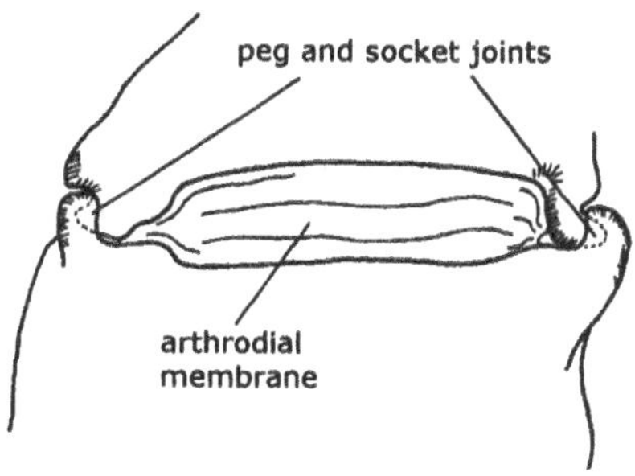

Fig. 1.2 Articulation in the crab, by means of water-lubricated peg-and-socket joints (after ref. 6)

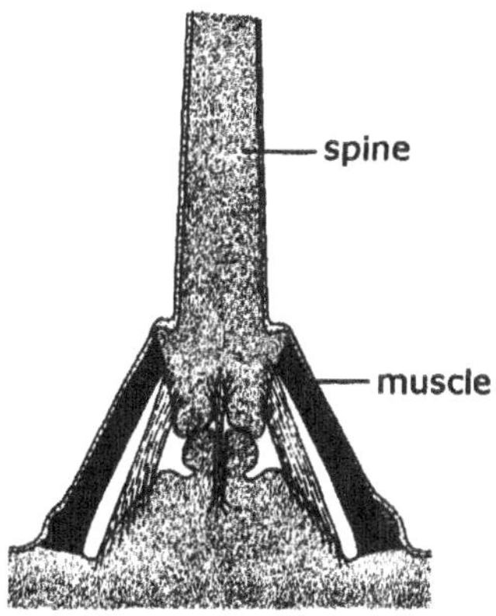

Fig. 1.3 The spine of a sea-urchin articulates relative to the body via a ball-and-socket joint with calcite bearing surfaces (after ref. 7)

1.3 Tribology of human joints – natural, and artificial

We may think of the synovial joints of the human body mainly in the context of the joints of the limb-bones, but the structure and function of this type of joint is more widespread. Even the very small auditory ossicles in the middle ear, the smallest bones in the body, have articulations which are 'typical synovial joints.... (The) articular surfaces are covered with articular cartilage and each joint is enveloped by a capsule containing much elastic tissue and lined by synovial membrane' **(8)**. The tribology of synovial joints in vertebrate limbs has been studied for many years, with early work by Osborne Reynolds (in 1886) suggesting that their lubrication involved the separation of the bearing surfaces by a continuous film of synovial fluid.

The development of successful hip prostheses following the pioneering work of McKee, Watson-Farrar, and Charnley in the 1950s has stimulated a large amount of research into the tribology of artificial and natural joints. Studies of joint lubrication recently reviewed by Unsworth **(9)**, and Dowson **(10, 11)** have provided comprehensive overviews of the lubrication of both natural and prosthetic joints, and of the important topic of wear in the latter. It is now clear that the thickness of the fluid film present in a hip prosthesis, to take an important example, depends critically on the mechanical properties of the materials of the bearing surfaces, as well as on their precise geometry and dimensions and on the applied load and sliding speed. Manufacturing tolerances and surface finish also have a profound effect on the regime of lubrication: whether in the terms familiar to tribologists, we have full film lubrication (in which the sliding surfaces are separated by a fluid film that is thick in comparison to the roughness of the surfaces), or boundary lubrication (in which the surfaces are separated only by lubricant molecules chemically attached to one or both surfaces), or the intermediate case of mixed lubrication. These regimes of lubrication result in markedly different values of friction (as shown in the classic Stribeck curve in Fig. 1.4) and wear rate.

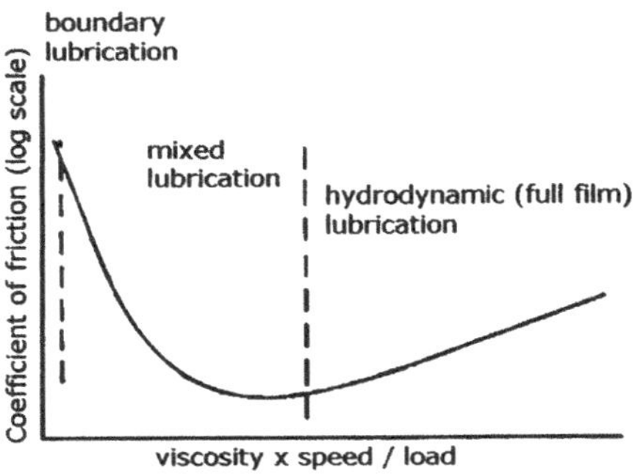

Fig. 1.4 The Stribeck curve which relates the coefficient of friction in a lubricated sliding contact to the applied load, sliding speed and the viscosity of the lubricant

For the hip prosthesis, only four broad material combinations have so far found favour in practical use: a metallic femoral head in a polymeric acetabular cup; a ceramic head in a polymeric cup; a ceramic head in a ceramic cup; and a metallic head in a metallic cup. Even within these classes there is little variation in the actual materials used, perhaps because of regulatory constraints or sheer conservatism, but more probably because these combinations have been found under many conditions to offer the potential for long-lived and reliable prostheses. The metal used for bearing surfaces is usually a cobalt-chromium-molybdenum alloy; the polymer ultra-high-molecular weight polyethylene (UHMWPE); and the ceramic high purity alumina, or in the case of ceramic-on-polymer joints only, in some cases partially stabilized zirconia. To the engineering tribologist with no exposure to the field of biotribology the success of these combinations appears surprising, and it is worth asking why they provide such good performance.

The use of polymers such as polytetrafluoroethylene (PTFE) and linear-chain polyethylenes (including UHMWPE) as bearing surfaces sliding against hard counterfaces is well established in engineering, and they are often incorporated into composite 'dry' (i.e. nominally unlubricated) bearings **(12)**. However, the low friction and wear which results from these materials is associated with the formation of a molecularly oriented film of polymer transferred to the counterface, which would be destroyed by two features which are both present in the hip joint: water, and motion which involves some relative rotation rather than purely linear sliding. It would seem that it is only the presence of significant fluid-film lubrication, as found in a hip prosthesis with closely conforming surfaces and a rather low bearing pressure (of a few MPa), that allows this combination to function as well as it does. One might even suggest that Charnley's innovative choice of a metallic femoral head sliding against a polymeric acetabular cup (initially PTFE but subsequently UHMWPE) was undoubtedly inspired, but probably for the wrong reasons.

Despite the success of the metal-on-polymer hip prosthesis, with low friction and relatively low wear rate, the polymeric wear debris produced during use over a period of years causes adverse pathological reaction in the surrounding tissues which is a frequent cause of osteolysis and joint loosening. The reduction of wear rate in order to minimize this effect is one of the most important challenges currently facing the biotribologist. An impressive reduction in the wear of UHMWPE in hip prostheses can be achieved by crosslinking the polymer chains **(13)**; the effect is much greater than the reduction which can be achieved by using a very smooth ceramic femoral head instead of metal **(10, 14)**. However, even lower wear rates can be achieved in metal-on-metal or ceramic-on-ceramic prostheses. The design of such joints, in particular metal-on-metal joints, appears at first sight to be surprising as it is often taken as axiomatic that in order to minimize wear in a tribological couple, the two sliding surfaces in contact should be of different alloys **(15)**. As in the case of the metal-on-polymer prosthesis, it is likely that the very low wear rates which can be achieved with such combinations are due to the presence of thin but nevertheless essential films of lubricant, and that these are favoured, and significant asperity contact is avoided, by the maintenance of extremely smooth surfaces and very small clearances (which are however sufficient to avoid seizure). Dowson has shown **(10)** how bearing clearances of a few tens of micrometres can lead to elastohydrodynamic film thicknesses of the order of tens of nanometres, which in the context of surfaces with roughnesses of the order of 10 nm leads to very low wear. The importance of precision in both manufacturing processes and metrology in order to achieve such results is evident.

1.4 Conclusions

The engineering tribologist has much to contribute to these aspects of biotribology, as the well-developed mechanical theories of lubrication can readily be applied to understanding the development and maintenance of the vital lubricant film within prostheses. The materials scientist can assist with an understanding of the relationship between the processing and microstructure of the materials used and their mechanical and other properties, as well as the important question of the formation of tribochemical surface films. However, as practitioners in the field are well aware, these aspects are by no means the whole story. The response of the body to the presence of a foreign prosthesis, and also to the production of wear debris, as well as the formation, nature and properties of the surface films formed in the sliding contact *in vivo* are all vitally important to the successful function of a prosthetic joint. Advances in the biotribology of prosthetic joints will require a special blend of understanding of such biological and biochemical topics, as well as of more conventional tribology.

References

(1) Oxford English Dictionary (with supplements, on-line edition) (2002); Merriam-Webster Collegiate Dictionary (on-line edition) (2002).

(2) **Dowson, D.** and **Wright, V.**, in The Rheology of Lubricants, Davenport, T. C. (ed.), Applied Science Publishers, Barking, pp. 81–88, 1973, cited by Dowson, D., History of Tribology, Longman, London, 1979.

(3) **Berry, R. M.**, Phil. Trans Roy. Soc. Lond. B 355 (2000) 503–509, 'Theories of rotary motors'.

(4) **Berg, H. C.**, Phil. Trans Roy. Soc. Lond. B 355 (2000) 491–501, 'Constraints on models for the flagellar rotary motor'.

(5) **Nakano, T.**, **Momozono, S.**, and **Aizawa, S.**, Synposes of Int. Tribology Conf., Nagasaki, Japan, 2000, 292, 'Tribological analysis of bacterial flagellar motor'.

(6) **Currey, J. D.**, Animal Skeletons, Arnold, London, 1970.

(7) **Smith, A.**, Echinoid Palaeobiology, George Allen and Unwin, 1984.

(8) Gray's Anatomy, Churchill Livingstone, Edinburgh, 1995.

(9) **Unsworth, A.**, Tribology International, 28 (1995) 485–495, 'Recent developments in the tribology of artificial joints'.

(10) **Dowson, D.**, Wear 190 (1995) 171–183, 'A comparative study of the performance of metallic and ceramic femoral head components in total replacement hip joints'.

(11) **Dowson, D.**, Institution of Mechanical Engineers, James Clayton Memorial Lecture, 2000, 'New joints for the millennium: wear control in total replacement hip joints'

(12) **Hutchings, I. M.**, Tribology: Friction and Wear of Engineering Materials, Arnold, London, 1992.

(13) **Wang, A.** *et al.*, Tribology International 31 (1998) 17–33, 'Lubrication and wear of ultra-high molecular weight polyethylene in total joint replacements'.

(14) **Unsworth, A.** *et al.*, in Thinning Films and Tribological Interfaces, Dowson, D. *et al.* eds., Tribology Series 38, Elsevier, 2000, 195–202, 'Tribology of replacement hip joints'.

(15) **Rabinowicz, E.**, Friction and Wear of Materials, 2nd ed., Wiley Interscience, 1995.

I M Hutchings
Department of Engineering, University of Cambridge, UK

2

Wear and Functional Biological Activity of Wear Debris Generated from UHMWPE-on-Zirconia Ceramic, Metal-on-Metal, and Alumina Ceramic-on-Ceramic Hip Prostheses During Hip Simulator Testing

J L Tipper, J B Matthews, E Ingham, T D Stewart, J Fisher, and **M H Stone**

Abstract

There is currently much interest in the characterization of wear debris from different types of hip-joint prostheses. There have been numerous studies on the wear of UHMWPE in hip-joint simulators, but relatively few studies on the wear of alternative materials such as metal-on-metal and ceramic-on-ceramic. The aim of this study was to compare the wear volumes and the functional biological activity (FBA) of the wear debris generated from zirconia ceramic-on-UHMWPE, cobalt–chrome metal-on-metal, and alumina ceramic-on-ceramic hip joints under standard and micro-separation simulation conditions in the same hip-joint simulator.

All prostheses showed a higher 'bedding in' wear rate, which was followed by a lower steady-state wear rate. Under standard simulation conditions, the zirconia ceramic-on-UHMWPE prostheses showed the highest wear rates (31 ±4.0 mm^3/million cycles), followed by the metal-on-metal (1.23 ±0.5 mm^3/million cycles), with the alumina ceramic-on-ceramic prostheses showing significantly (p<0.01) lower wear rates at 0.05 ±0.02 mm^3/million cycles. The alumina ceramic-on-ceramic wear rate was 10–50-fold lower than some clinical retrieval studies, and the wear stripe observed on retrieved components was not reproduced under standard simulation conditions. The mean (±95 per cent confidence limits) size of the UHMWPE wear debris was 300 ±200 nm (range 0.1–50 μm), 30 ±2.25 nm (range 9–66 nm) for the metal particles, and 9 ±0.5 nm (range 2–27 nm) for the alumina–ceramic wear particles. The UHMWPE and cobalt–chrome wear particles were similar to those described *in vivo*; however, alumina–ceramic particles up to 3 μm have been identified in periprosthetic tissues from around ceramic-on-ceramic prostheses.

When micro-separation of the alumina–ceramic components was introduced into the simulation, clinically relevant wear rates, wear patterns, and wear particles were generated. The wear rate increased to 1.84 ±0.3 mm^3/million cycles and the stripe wear feature was reproduced on the alumina femoral heads. In addition to the nanometre-sized wear particles generated under standard simulation conditions, larger micrometre-sized alumina wear particles were also observed.

The FBA of the wear particles was determined by integrating measurements from *in vitro* wear simulations, particle characterization, and *in vitro* cell culture studies. These studies revealed that the UHMWPE particles produced in this study demonstrated a three-fold higher specific biological activity and a 50-fold higher FBA than the alumina–ceramic particles generated under micro-separation simulation conditions.

This study revealed significant differences in the wear volumes, size distributions, and FBAof the wear particles generated from the three different prostheses under clinically relevant conditions in *in vitro* wear simulations.

2.1 Introduction

Aseptic loosening is the primary cause of failure of total hip replacements (THRs), and accounts for almost three-quarters of all revision operations **(1)**. It has been linked with osteolysis induced by ultra-high molecular weight polyethylene (UHMWPE) wear debris **(2–6)**. The occurrence and severity of osteolysis appear to be related to the size and volume concentration of wear particles released **(7)**. By lowering the quantity and generation rate of wear particles, the occurrence of long-term aseptic loosening should therefore be reduced. The majority of THRs performed in the UK comprise a metal femoral head manufactured from either cobalt–chrome or stainless steel, articulating on an UHMWPE acetabular cup. Scratch damage to metal femoral heads has been shown to increase the wear rate of UHMWPE *in vivo* and during *in vitro* testing **(8, 9)**. It was therefore assumed that the introduction of scratch-resistant ceramic femoral heads would lower the wear rate of UHMWPE and thus have a beneficial effect on osteolysis. Alumina and zirconia femoral heads articulating on UHMWPE acetabular cups were introduced into clinical practice in 1975, and the resulting *in vivo* wear rates of UHMWPE acetabular cups have since been shown to be 50 per cent lower than UHMWPE-on-metal articulations **(10)**. In addition, alumina femoral heads have demonstrated lower UHMWPE wear and increased resistance to scratching *in vitro* **(11)**.

As the problems associated with UHMWPE wear particles have become more apparent, interest in alternative bearing material combinations, such as metal-on-metal (MOM) and ceramic-on-ceramic (COC) prostheses, has increased. Some of the first-generation McKee-Farrar MOM hip prostheses performed well for 20 years or more **(12)**, and the wear rate of first-generation MOM hip prostheses was reported to be 1–6 mm^3 per year, compared with 30–100 mm^3 for traditional metal-on-polyethylene hips **(13–15)**. These favourable clinical results led to the introduction of second-generation MOM hip prostheses, which are superior in terms of both design and materials. These have demonstrated low wear rates when compared with metal-on-polyethylene in *in vitro* testing **(16)**, and short-term clinical performance has been encouraging, with reports of mean wear rates as low as 0.3 mm^3 per year **(17–21)**. The suitability of new materials and designs has traditionally been assessed on wear volume alone; however, a low wear volume is not the only important factor governing the long-term clinical outcome of a total hip replacement. The size, morphology, and biological reactivity of any wear particles released are all equally important.

Recent studies have shown that the wear particles generated in MOM hip prostheses are in the nanometre size range **(22–24)**. Consequently, the number of particles produced in a MOM articulation may exceed the number of UHMWPE particles produced by a metal-on-polyethylene articulation, despite the low wear volume of the MOM prosthesis. Doorn *et al.* **(22)** isolated and characterized metal wear particles from the periprosthetic tissues from first- and second-generation MOM hip prostheses. The particles were in the size range 51–116 nm, and were mainly round in shape. These authors estimated that between 6.7×10^{12} and 2.5×10^{14} particles would be produced per year, 13–500 times more particles than the 5×10^{11} UHMWPE particles produced per year in a typical metal-on-polyethylene prosthesis **(22)**. The small size of the particles gives rise to large numbers of particles, even for wear volumes as low as 1 mm^3 per year. In addition, there is concern over the distribution of these small particles around the body and the biological effects that they may have on cells and tissues. Metal particles have been shown to be disseminated throughout the body and have been found in the lymph nodes, liver, spleen, and bone marrow **(25–28)**. Little is known about their long-term systemic effects, although concerns about metal sensitivity **(29)** and increased incidence of haematological cancers, such as lymphoma and leukaemia, have been raised **(30)**.

It is still not clear whether osteolysis occurs around MOM hip prostheses. In general, the new generation MOM prostheses have not been associated with particle-induced osteolysis. More recently, however, a report by Beaulé *et al.* **(31)** described osteolysis in association with a MOM prosthesis induced by joint fluid access to the effective joint space. In addition, the results of long-term implantation are at present unknown. Schmalzried *et al.* **(32)** studied a series of first-generation McKee-Farrar hips, some of which had been implanted for 30 years, and found the incidence of osteolysis to be four per cent for the whole series. This compared favourably with metal-on-polyethylene hips, but indicated that MOM prostheses may not eliminate osteolysis in the longer term. In general, histological studies of periprosthetic tissues have not shown an inflammatory reaction to metal wear particles, but areas of tissue necrosis have been associated with visible metal particles **(20, 22, 33)**. There have been many studies on the effect of micrometre-sized metal wear particles on cells *in vitro* **(34–37)**, but the effects of nanometre-sized particles have not been widely studied, and the relevance of the studies using the larger particles is debatable. Recent studies from our research group indicated that nanometre-sized metal wear particles were cytotoxic to primary human mononuclear cells and fibroblasts at elevated concentrations *in vitro* **(38)**. Nevertheless, the current second-generation MOM bearings are showing considerable potential as an osteolysis-free solution for younger patients.

Ceramic-on-ceramic hip prostheses have been used clinically for over 25 years. The wear rates of retrieved COC prostheses are generally much lower than those of metal-on-polyethylene bearings, and are in the order of 1 mm^3 per year **(39)**. However, occasional cases of more severe wear have been reported. Under ideal conditions in the laboratory, extremely low wear rates of 0.01–0.1 mm^3/million cycles have been reported **(40, 41)**, which are at least one order of magnitude lower than those reported *in vivo*. Attention has recently focused on understanding the differences between laboratory and *ex vivo* wear rates, and attempting to investigate the causes of severe wear in isolated cases *in vivo*. In an attempt to increase wear, *in vitro* wear simulations have utilized water as a lubricant, as opposed to bovine serum, to produce harsher lubrication conditions **(42)**. However, wear volumes remained well below those reported in the majority of retrieval cases. An increased angle of inclination of the acetabular cup has also been cited as a possible cause of accelerated wear of COC prostheses *in vivo* **(39)**. However, increasing the acetabular cup angle from 45 to 60 degrees did not significantly increase the wear rate *in vitro* **(43)**.

Recent examination of retrieved modern alumina-on-alumina hip prostheses, manufactured after 1995, revealed a small band of wear ('stripe' wear) around the rims of the acetabular cups **(44)**. This was the first evidence that modern alumina–alumina hip prostheses also exhibited the 'stripe' wear morphology frequently observed in retrieved first generation alumina–alumina prostheses **(39)**. Fluoroscopy studies have shown separation of the ball and socket during the swing phase of walking for metal-on-UHMWPE hip prostheses **(45)**. It has been suggested that this micro-separation of prosthesis components, as shown in Fig. 2.1, could occur in any hip prosthesis, and may be a factor involved in the initiation of 'stripe' wear observed on retrieved alumina COC hip prostheses. Nevelos *et al.* **(44)** introduced micro-separation of alumina COC hip prosthesis components into *in vitro* wear simulations, and reproduced clinically relevant wear rates, wear patterns, and mechanisms for the first time.

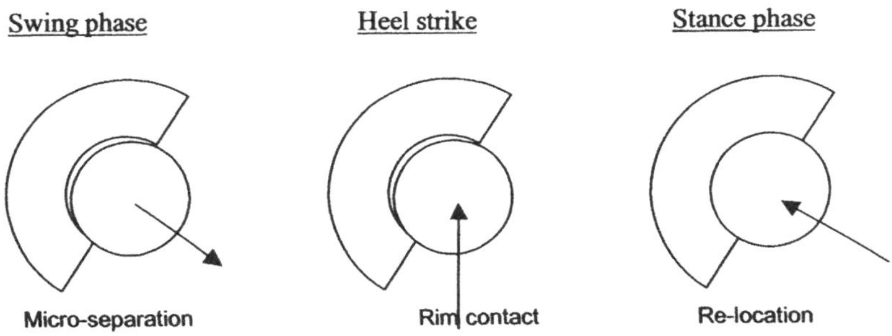

Fig. 2.1 Schematic illustration of micro-separation motion

Ceramic wear particles have been reported to be in the nanometre size range, but larger particles up to 7 μm have also been identified in *ex vivo* specimens **(46, 47)**. There is a limited amount of data available in the literature on the biological responses to ceramic wear particles. In its bulk form alumina is chemically inert, and this was one of the factors that influenced its selection as a bearing material. Recently, evidence of wear-debris-induced osteolysis has been reported in a series of alumina COC hip prostheses **(47)**. Histological examination of the periprosthetic tissues from around revised Mittelmeier hip prostheses revealed abundant ceramic wear debris with a mean size of 0.71 μm (range 0.13–7.2 μm). In addition, Hatton *et al.* **(48)** reported that alumina particles with a mean size of 0.5 ±0.19 μm (±SD) induced the production of the osteolytic cytokine TNF-α by peripheral blood mononuclear phagocytes *in vitro*, albeit at a reduced level to that produced in response to UHMWPE particles of a similar size and at the same concentration. To date, the biological activity of the nanometre-sized wear particles has not been determined. However, with *in vivo* wear rates of approximately 1 mm^3 per year, ceramic-on-ceramic couples also offer considerable potential as an osteolysis-free solution for young patients.

There have been a number of studies of polyethylene wear in hip-joint simulators **(49–56)**. However, different designs of simulator, together with the application of different loads and motions, mean that the results are often difficult to compare directly. In addition, relatively few studies on the wear of alternative materials such as metal-on-metal and ceramic-on-ceramic prostheses have been performed. To date, no direct comparison of the wear debris generated from these three different materials has been reported. The aim of this study was to compare the wear volumes and wear debris generated from zirconia ceramic-on-UHMWPE, MOM, and COC hip prostheses under identical conditions in a hip-joint simulator. However, it is important that wear simulations produce realistic clinically relevant wear particles, as well as clinically relevant wear rates and wear patterns. The alumina COC prostheses were therefore tested under standard and micro-separation simulation conditions. In addition, the aim of this study was to determine the FBA of clinically relevant wear particles produced from these different bearing materials in *in vitro* wear simulations.

2.2 Materials

Three types of hip prosthesis were studied: zirconia–ceramic femoral heads (Howmedica International) on UHMWPE GUR 1120 acetabular cups (γ irradiated with 2.5 Mrad in air); low-carbon (<0.07 per cent) wrought cobalt–chrome alloy (ASTM F1537) femoral heads on high-carbon (>0.2 per cent) wrought cobalt–chrome alloy (ASTM F1537) acetabular cups; medical grade HIPed 'BIOLOX Forte' alumina–ceramic femoral heads (CeramTec AG; ISO 6474) on medical grade HIPed 'BIOLOX Forte' alumina–ceramic (CeramTec AG; ISO 6474) acetabular cups. All prostheses had 28 mm diameter heads and a minimum of three prostheses of each type was tested.

2.3 Methods

2.3.1 Hip simulator testing

2.3.1.1 Standard simulator testing

The Leeds MKII physiological hip-joint simulator was used, which positions the cup in the superior position to the head and inclined in the anatomical position between 45 and 60 degrees to the vertical axis. A single-axis, twin-peak, Paul type loading curve **(57)** was applied through the vertical axis of the cup. Two directions of motion were applied: flexion–extension (+30 degrees and –15 degrees) and internal–external rotation (±10 degrees). The motions were 90 degrees out of phase such that an open elliptical wear track was generated between the components. These conditions have previously been shown to reproduce similar wear rates and features to those seen when three independently controlled loads and motions were applied to UHMWPE cups **(58)**. All simulator tests were performed at a frequency of 1 Hz in 25 per cent (v/v) bovine serum plus 0.1 per cent (w/v) sodium azide, which was added to retard bacterial growth.

For the MOM and alumina COC prostheses, wear volumes were determined gravimetrically every million cycles to five million cycles. Prior to weighing, the femoral heads and acetabular cups were cleaned with a mild detergent, followed by ultrasonic cleaning with isopropanol, to allow accurate measurement of wear and surface topography. The first million cycles represented 'bedding in' wear, as has been described previously for hard-on-hard bearings **(59, 60)**. For the UHMWPE-on-zirconia ceramic prostheses, changes in shape and volume of the acetabular cups were determined using a three-dimensional co-ordinate measurement machine (CMM; Kemco, UK). The volume changes due to both creep and wear were monitored every half million cycles up to five million cycles **(61)**. The surface roughness of the femoral heads was measured before and after testing using a contacting three-dimentional Form Talysurf (Taylor Hobson Limited, Leicester, UK) or non-contacting surface profilometry (UBM Messtechnik GmbH, Ettlingen, Germany). The initial surface roughness (R_a) was between 0.005 and 0.008 μm for all femoral heads, regardless of material. The diametral clearances of the MOM components were between 58 and 62 μm, and between 40 and 60 μm for the COC prostheses. In addition, the bearing surfaces of the alumina ceramic-on-ceramic prostheses were analysed using a WYKO NT2000 white light interferometer after two and five million cycles of simulator testing.

2.3.1.2 Micro-separation simulator testing

Three 28 mm 'BIOLOX forte' (HIPed) alumina ceramic-on-ceramic prosthesis were tested in the Leeds MKII six station hip simulator under simulation conditions that incorporated micro-separation. Micro-separation motion was achieved by applying a force of approximately 400 N to the acetabular cup holder in the medio-lateral direction using a spring. This force, combined with a low swing-phase load of <50 N, allowed the joint to separate. On heel strike, the head contacted the rim of the micro-displaced cup, before the joint relocated in the normal position during the stance phase. The force applied by the separation spring was regularly adjusted to produce between 300 and 500 μm of medio-lateral displacement throughout the study. The micro-separation simulations were performed in 25 per cent (v/v) bovine serum for five million cycles under a peak load of 2.2 kN. Wear was determined gravimetrically every million cycles, and after testing the worn areas of all components were analysed using Talysurf contacting profilometry and scanning electron microscopy (SEM).

Serum lubricants from all simulator tests were collected and stored at –20 °C until required for wear debris characterization.

2.3.2 Wear debris isolation and characterization

UHMWPE wear particles were isolated from wear test lubricants by digestion and observed using SEM. Alumina–ceramic and cobalt–chrome wear particles generated in standard wear simulations were characterized by transmission electron microscopy (TEM), and alumina–ceramic wear particles generated in micro-separation wear simulations were characterized by both SEM and TEM.

2.3.2.1 Isolation of UHMWPE wear debris

UHMWPE wear debris was isolated from the serum lubricants using a method described previously by Besong *et al.* **(62)**. Briefly, approximately 60 ml of serum lubricant was digested with 12 M potassium hydroxide for 48 h at 60 °C. Contaminating proteins and lipids were removed by the addition of an equal volume of chloroform:methanol (2:1) followed by centrifugation at 2000 g for 10 minutes at room temperature. Any remaining proteins were removed by precipitation with ice-cold absolute ethanol followed by centrifugation at 2000 g for 2 h at 4 °C. Polyethylene wear debris was recovered by sequential filtration on to pre-weighed 10 and 0.1 μm Cyclopore™ membranes (Whatman International, UK). The mass of debris on each filter was determined gravimetrically. A section of each filter was coated with gold and observed using SEM (Hitachi S700). Representative photographs were taken at magnifications of ×200–20 000.

2.3.2.2 *Characterization of cobalt–chrome and alumina–ceramic wear particles by TEM*

Cobalt–chrome and alumina–ceramic wear particles were characterized by TEM. An appropriate volume of serum (60–100 ml) was centrifuged (12 000 g, 10 minutes, 4 °C) to pellet the wear particles and the supernatant was discarded. The pellet was then fixed in 2.5 per cent (v/v) glutaraldehyde in phosphate buffered saline (PBS) at pH 7.4 for 2 h at 4 °C. The samples were washed three times in PBS for 2 h at 4°C, and fixed in 1 per cent (w/v) osmium tetraoxide for 1–2 h at 4 °C. Residual osmium tetraoxide was removed by washing in PBS for 15 minutes and the samples were then dehydrated through graded ethanols [70, 90, and 100 per cent (v/v)] at room temperature for 10–20 minutes. The samples were polymerized in araldite resin for 20–24 h at 70 °C and 100 nm sections were cut using an LKB ultramicrotome fitted with a diamond knife. The sections were transferred to copper grids for staining with lead nitrate and sodium citrate for 1–2 minutes. The samples were double stained with 15 per cent (v/v) uranyl acetate. The sections were then observed using a Jeol 1200 EX transmission electron microscope and representative photographs of the wear debris were taken at magnifications of ×25–75 000. The presence of cobalt, chromium, or aluminium was confirmed by energy dispersive X-ray (EDX) analysis (Link Isis, Oxford Instruments).

2.3.2.3 *Characterization of alumina–ceramic wear particles by SEM*

Wear particles were collected by centrifugation of wear test lubricants at 2000 g for 20 minutes, followed by washing three times with PBS to remove proteins. Wear particles were resuspended in pyrogen-free water (Baxter Healthcare). The ceramic wear particles were dispersed by sonication at 250 W for 2–3 minutes and then collected by filtration on to filter membranes with 15 nm pores (Nucleopore™). A section of the filter was mounted on an aluminum stub and coated with gold before being observed using a Hitachi S700 SEM. Images of the ceramic wear particles were captured digitally using Image Slave™ at magnifications between ×200 and ×10 000. The presence of aluminium was confirmed using a scanning electron microscope fitted with EDX analysis equipment (Link Isis, Oxford Instruments).

2.3.2.4 *Image analysis of wear particles*

All wear particles were characterized using digital image analysis (Image Pro Plus, Media Cybernetics, USA). The UHMWPE wear particles were analysed quantitatively. The percentage frequency and area distributions of the particles were determined as a function of particle size, r, in three different size ranges 0.1–1.0 μm, 1.0–10 μm, and 10–100 μm. Assuming a constant particle thickness of 0.4 μm on the 0.1 μm filter, a volume distribution was determined **(62)**. Cobalt–chrome and alumina–ceramic wear particles were characterized using mean maximum diameter or length measurements. A minimum of 100 particles per sample were measured by image analysis. Statistical analysis of the results was carried out using single classification analysis of variance (ANOVA), and comparison of minimum significant differences by the T-method.

2.3.3 Determination of biological activity of wear particles

The FBA of wear particles was achieved by integrating measurements from *in vitro* wear simulations, particle characterization, and *in vitro* cell culture studies **(63)**.

The biological activity function *B*(*r*) of *in vitro* generated sterile endotoxin-free UHMWPE wear debris was determined as a function of particle size (*r*) at fixed volume concentrations. Particles were co-cultured for 24 h with primary human mononuclear phagocytes isolated from the peripheral blood of three healthy volunteers by density centrifugation (Lymphoprep, Nycomed Pharma AS Diagnostics, Norway). Tumour necrosis factor-alpha (TNF-α) was used as a marker for biological activity, as it has been shown to be one of the major osteolytic mediators released in response to clinically relevant UHMWPE wear particles **(64)**. In addition, TNF-α has been shown to correlate with bone resorption **(65, 66)**. TNF-α production in response to UHMWPE particles at a concentration of 10 and 100 μm^3 debris per cell was measured by double antibody sandwich ELISA as described previously **(64)**. All tests were performed in triplicate using cells cultured without particles as a negative control and cells stimulated with 2 $\mu g\ ml^{-1}$ lipopolysaccharide as a positive control. The viability of the cells was determined by the MTT assay. Culture supernatants were assayed for TNF-α production and results expressed as specific activity to normalize for variations in cell number and/or cell viability. Levels of cytokine in particle-stimulated cultures were compared with negative controls by one-way ANOVA and calculation of the minimum significant difference (MSD) using the T-method. Biological activity was determined in three particle size ranges, 0.1–1.0 μm, 1–10 μm, and 10–100 μm at 100 μm^3 debris per cell and normalized with respect to the lowest size range.

The TNF-α response to alumina–ceramic wear particles generated under micro-separation simulation conditions was also determined. Alumina–ceramic wear particles were removed from the serum lubricants by centrifugation at 2000 g for 20 minutes. Wear particles were heat treated at 180 °C for 4 h to remove contaminating endotoxin, and co-cultured with peripheral blood mononuclear cells isolated from healthy volunteers at 100 μm^3 debris per mononuclear phagocyte as described by Hatton *et al.* **(48)**. All tests were performed in triplicate and controls were as described for the UHMWPE study above.

Volumetric wear volumes were determined for each of the prosthesis types under standard simulation conditions and micro-separation conditions (alumina ceramic-on-ceramic only) as described above. Wear particles were characterized by size, mass, and morphology by the methods described above in Section 3.2.4, and the volumetric concentration *C*(*r*) of particles as a function of size was determined. The specific biological activity (SBA) index (biological activity per unit volume) was determined by integrating the product of the biological activity function [*B*(*r*)] and the volumetric concentration [*C*(*r*)] of particles in each size range. The FBA index was defined as the product of the volumetric wear rate ($mm^3/10^6$cycles) and SBA.

2.4 Results

2.4.1 Standard wear simulation conditions

The wear scars on the heads and cups for the zirconia-on-UHMWPE and MOM prostheses were located in the superior quadrant, as found clinically. The majority of the wear for the metal-on-metal articulations occurred on the low-carbon, cobalt–chrome heads. Some deep scratches (>1 μm) were observed on the low carbon heads, possibly caused by carbides which were present in the high carbon cups. A thin layer of calcium phosphate deposit was observed on all components from the MOM pairings, which made accurate surface analysis by contacting profilometry difficult. No change in surface roughness was detected for the alumina–ceramic components tested under standard simulation conditions, and very few wear features were observed using three-dimensional contacting profilometry. However, when the wear surfaces were subjected to closer inspection using a WYKO NT2000 white light interferometer, small scale pitting and short curved scratches were visible in the contact areas of both heads and cups The pitting may have been caused by small-scale grain removal, and the scratches by third body wear. Polishing marks from manufacture were also visible on the surfaces. The zirconia–ceramic heads also remained undamaged after testing. Scanning electron microscopy of the worn surfaces of the UHMWPE cups revealed areas of localized adhesive wear and fatigue damage. The volumetric wear rates for the three materials are shown in Table 2.1. The initial 'bedding in' wear was always higher than the steady-state wear for each type of prosthesis. For the UHMWPE cups the initial 'bedding in' wear also included creep deformation. The zirconia ceramic-on-UHMWPE had the highest steady-state wear rate at 31 mm^3/million cycles, and the alumina ceramic-on-ceramic (standard simulation conditions) the lowest at 0.05 mm^3/million cycles. There was at least one order of magnitude difference between the wear rates of the different prosthesis types, which was highly significant ($p<0.01$).

Table 2.1 Volumetric wear rates of the three prosthesis types

Material combination	*Wear rate (mm^3/million cycles) ±95% confidence limits*	
	Bedding in	*Steady state*
Zirconia-on-UHMWPE	53	31 ±4.0
Cobalt–chrome-on-cobalt–chrome	3.1	1.23 ±0.5
Alumina-on-alumina (std.)	0.11 ±0.05	0.05 ±0.02
Alumina-on-alumina (μsep)	4.0 ±0.6	1.3 ±0.3

std., standard simulation conditions; μsep, micro-separation simulation conditions.

2.4.2 Micro-separation wear simulation testing

Wear rates are summarized in Table 2.1, and Fig. 2.2. When alumina ceramic-on-ceramic couples were subjected to micro-separation simulation conditions the wear rates increased dramatically compared to standard simulation conditions. Under standard simulation conditions the bedding in (0–1 million cycles) wear rate was 0.11 ±0.05 mm^3/million cycles and the steady state (1–5 million cycles) wear rate was 0.05 ±0.02 mm^3/million cycles. Under micro-separation simulation conditions, the bedding in wear rate increased to 4.0 ±0.6 mm^3/million cycles and steady state wear increased to 1.3 ±0.3 mm^3/million cycles. This was significantly higher than under standard simulation conditions and resulted in an overall wear rate of 1.84 ±0.3 mm^3/million cycles, which was similar to the average *ex vivo* wear rates of well fixed alumina COC prostheses at 1–5 mm^3/year. 'Stripe' wear on the femoral heads was initiated during the first million cycles (bedding in). This stripe wear increased surface roughness R_a from <0.01 μm to between 0.14 and 0.3 μm. Scanning electron microscopy revealed intergranular fracture [Fig. 2.3(a)] similar to that observed with retrieved alumina ceramic-on-ceramic prostheses [Fig. 2.3(b)]. Corresponding surface changes on the rim of the acetabular cups were also observed under micro-separation simulation conditions.

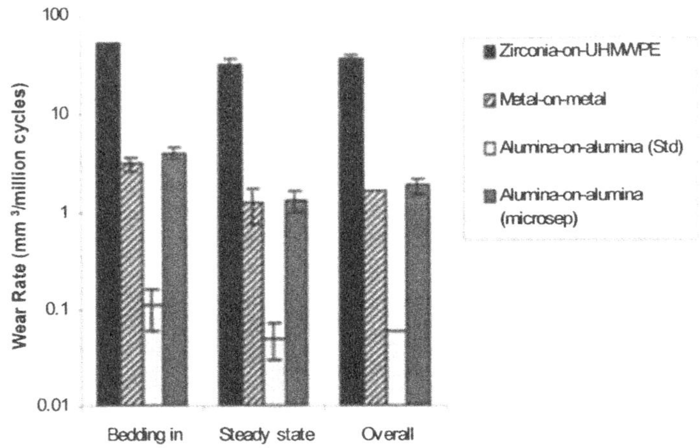

Fig. 2.2 Average wear rates for the different prosthesis types over the different stages of the wear simulation

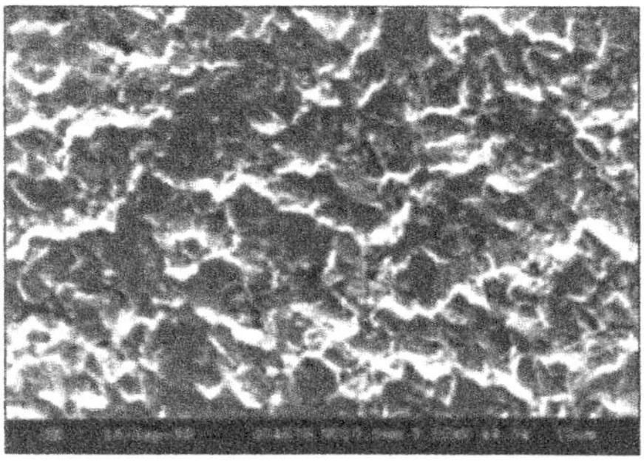

(a) in the centre of the wear stripe on an alumina–ceramic femoral head tested *in vitro* under micro-separation simulation (SEM image, bar 10 μm)

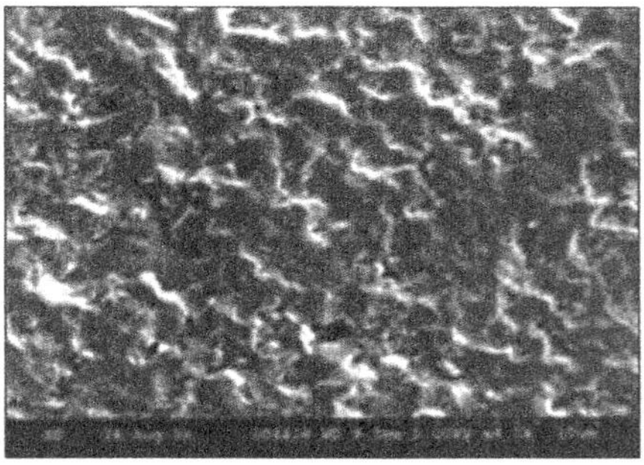

(b) on a retrieved alumina–ceramic femoral head (SEM image, bar 10 μm)

Fig. 2.3 Intergranular fracture of the alumina–ceramic observed

2.4.3 Characterization of the wear particles from the three prosthesis types

Wear particles larger than 100 nm for UHMWPE and larger than 2 nm for the metal-on-metal and alumina ceramic-on-ceramic prostheses were successfully characterized. The mean (±95 per cent confidence limits) sizes of the debris were 300 ±200 nm for the UHMWPE particles, 30 ±2.25 nm for the metal particles, and 9 ±0.5 nm for the alumina–ceramic wear particles generated under standard simulation conditions. The UHMWPE particles were significantly larger ($p<0.05$) than both the metal and ceramic particles, and the metal particles were significantly larger than the ceramic particles ($p<0.05$). The UHMWPE particles generated in the zirconia ceramic-on-UHMWPE articulations and characterized by SEM are shown in Figs 2.4(a) and 2.4(b). Metal and ceramic particles characterized by TEM are shown in Fig. 2.5(a)–(d). One of the most striking differences between the wear particles generated in the different prosthesis types was that the UHMWPE wear particles ranged in size from 100 to 50 000 nm. UHMWPE particles were not detected below 100 nm, but particles in this size range may exist, even though the techniques currently employed in the isolation of UHMWPE wear particles from serum and tissues do not allow their isolation. A variety of particle morphologies were observed from submicrometre granules [Fig. 2.4(a)] to large flakes or shards above 50 μm in size [Fig. 2.4(b)].

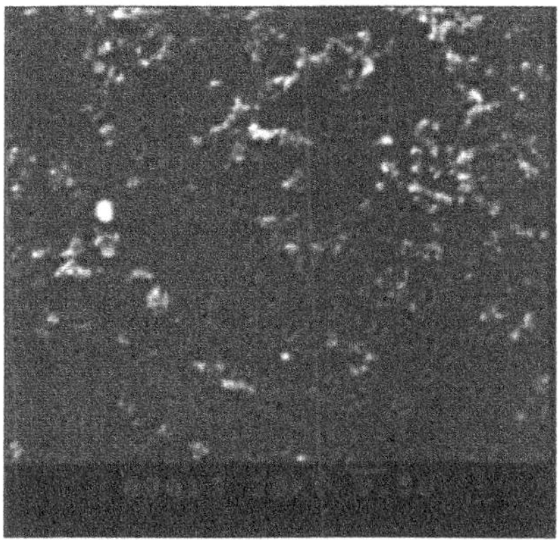

(a) Sub-micrometre granules of UHMWPE isolated on a 0.1 μm filter membrane, bar 0.5 μm

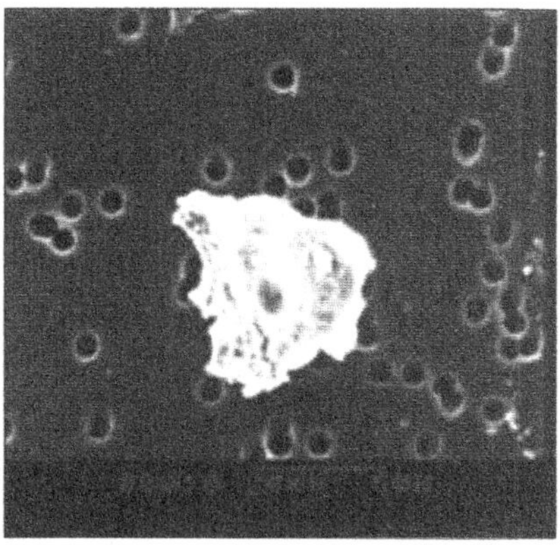

(b) A large flake-like particle isolated on the 10 μm filter membrane, bar 50 μm

Fig. 2.4 UHMWPE wear particles generated from the zirconia ceramic-on-UHMWPE prostheses in the hip simulator (SEM images)

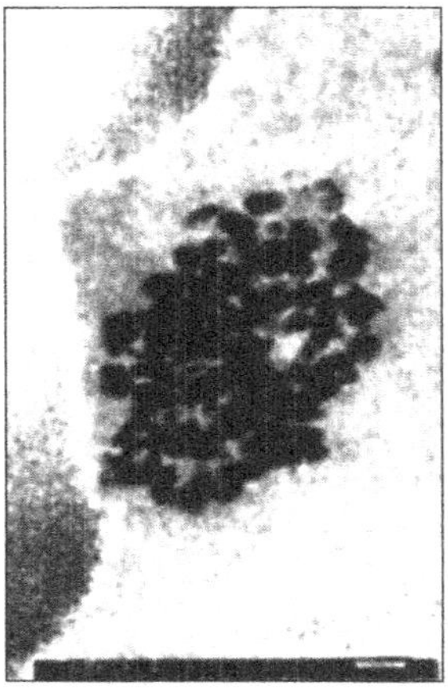

(a) Nanometre-sized cobalt–chromium wear particles generated from the metal-on-metal articulations (TEM image, bar 100 nm)

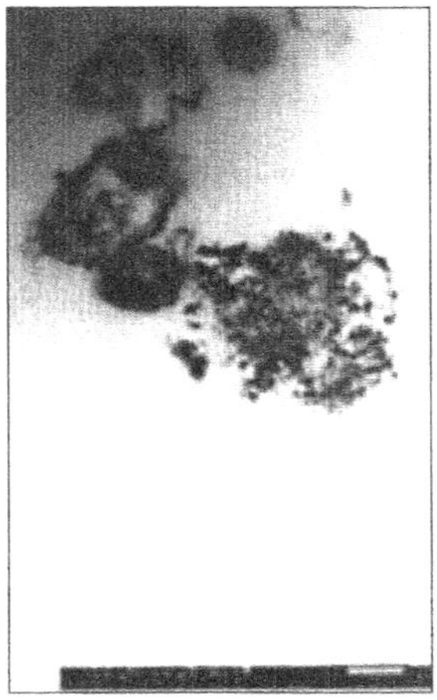

(b) Nanometre-sized alumina–ceramic wear particles generated from the alumina ceramic-on-ceramic articulations under standard simulation conditions (TEM image, bar 200 nm)

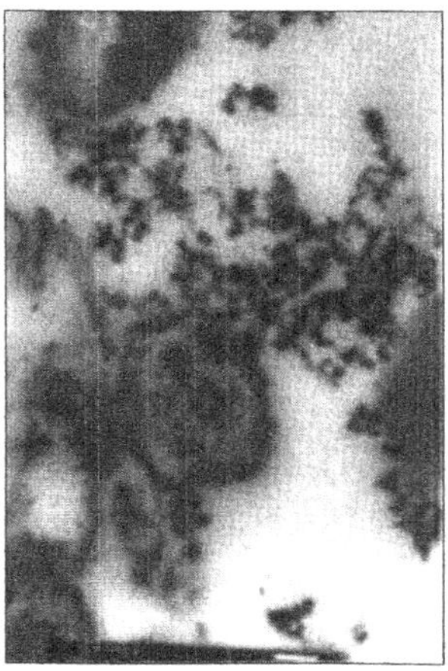

(c) Nanometre-sized alumina–ceramic wear particles generated from the alumina ceramic-on-ceramic articulations under micro-separation simulation conditions (TEM image, bar 100 nm)

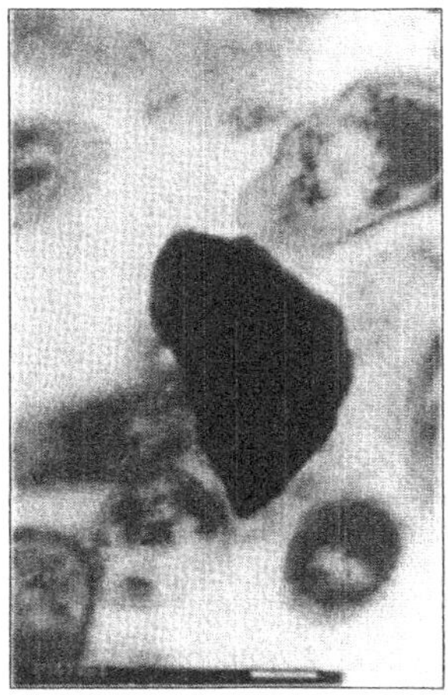

(d) Micrometre-sized alumina–ceramic wear particles generated from the alumina ceramic-on-ceramic articulations under micro-separation simulation conditions (TEM image, bar 100 nm)

Fig. 2.5 Wear particles generated in the hip-joint simulator wear tests from the hard-on-hard bearings

In contrast, the wear particles generated under standard simulation conditions in both the MOM and COC couples were very uniform in both size and morphology. The metal particles were 30 ±5 nm (range 9–66 nm) in size, and the majority were oval to round in shape and appeared as electron dense aggregates or clumps of particles [shown in Fig. 2.5(a)]. The particles generated in the COC couples under standard simulation conditions were even smaller at 9 ±0.5 nm (range 2–27.5 nm) and were also oval to round in appearance. These particles also appeared as electron dense aggregates when viewed using TEM [Fig. 2.5(b)].

However, when micro-separation was introduced into the simulation, a bimodal distribution of particles was produced. In addition to the nanometre-sized particles (4–100 nm), larger micrometre-sized (0.1–3 μm) particles were produced under micro-separation testing. The majority of the small alumina–ceramic particles characterized by TEM from micro-separation testing were oval to round in shape and appeared as electron dense aggregates [Fig. 2.5(c)]. The larger wear particles generated under micro-separation testing were polygonal in shape [Fig. 2.5(d)]. Serum lubricants from micro-separation were also analysed by SEM, which revealed many larger polygonal micrometre-sized particles [Fig. 2.6(a)] as well as aggregates of smaller submicrometre-sized particles [Fig. 2.6(b)].

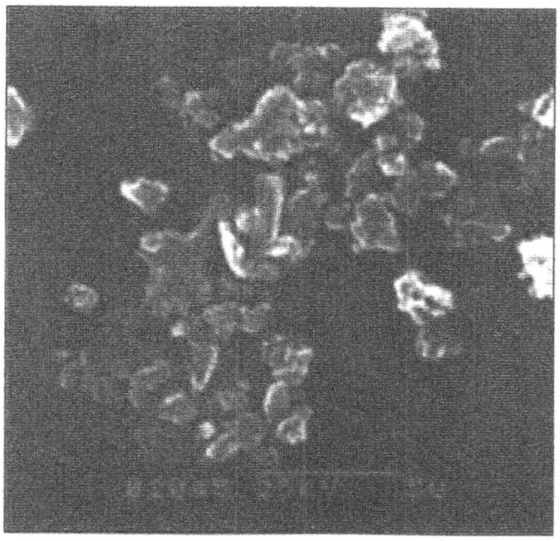

(a) Micrometre-sized polygonal alumina–ceramic particles generated from alumina ceramic-on-ceramic hip prostheses, bar 5 μm

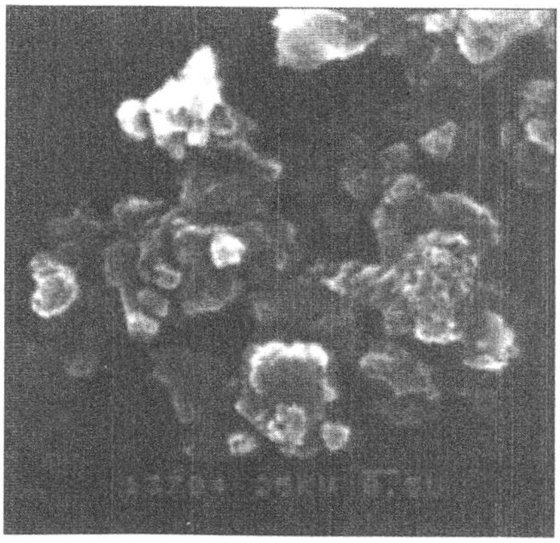

(b) Sub-micrometre-sized alumina–ceramic particles generated from alumina ceramic-on-ceramic hip prostheses, bar 0.5 μm

Fig. 2.6 Alumina–ceramic wear particles generated under micro-separation conditions and observed by SEM

The wear particles from the UHMWPE-on-zirconia–ceramic were quantitatively analysed. The mode of the frequency distribution of particle size was in the 0.1–1.0 μm size range, with 96 per cent of the particles in this range (Fig. 2.7). The mass distribution with respect to particle size is shown in Fig. 2.8. The majority of the mass, 73 ±2.42 per cent (mean ±SE) was composed of particles that were smaller than 10 μm in size.

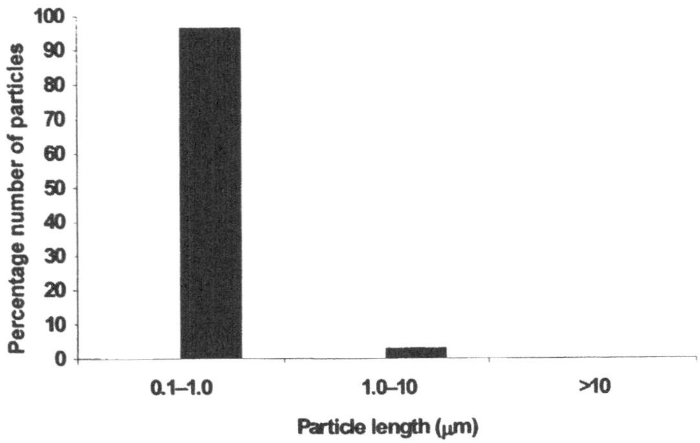

Fig. 2.7 Frequency distribution (mean ±SE) of the UHMWPE particles generated in the zirconia ceramic-on-UHMWPE articulations in the hip joint simulator – less than 0.1 per cent of the particles were >10 μm in length, and therefore were not included

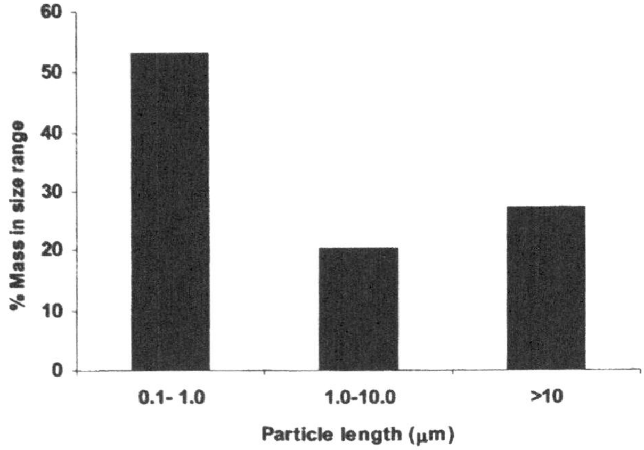

Fig. 2.8 Mass distribution (mean ±SE) of the UHMWPE particles as a function of size generated in the zirconia ceramic-on-UHMWPE articulations in the hip joint simulator

2.4.4 Functional biological activity (FBA) of the wear particles from the different prosthesis types

The biological activity index as a function of particle size $B(r)$ is shown in Table 2.2. The most biologically active UHMWPE particle size range (0.1–1.0 μm) was assigned a value of unity for each donor volunteer, hence normalizing the data to remove inter-donor variability. The particles in the 1.0–10 μm size range were five times less active than the particles in the

0.1–1.0 μm size range, and the particles in the 10–100 μm size range were 25-fold less active than the smallest particles (Table 2.2). The biological activity of nanometre-sized cobalt–chrome particles from MOM prostheses remains to be determined, as does the activity of nanometre-sized alumina wear particles generated from alumina ceramic-on-ceramic prostheses under standard simulation conditions. The majority of the alumina–ceramic particles generated in the ceramic-on-ceramic prostheses under micro-separation simulation conditions were between 4 nm and 1 μm in size. The biological activity of the alumina–ceramic particles was five times lower than that of UHMWPE particles of a similar size (Table 2.2). The volumetric concentrations of the particles as a function of size are shown in Table 2.3 for the different prosthesis types. Approximately 53 per cent of the UHMWPE particles were in the smallest size range, and 100 per cent of the wear particles from both the MOM and COC prostheses were between 0.1 and 1.0 μm (Table 2.3).

Table 2.2 Biological activity index *B*(*r*) for wear particles from the different prosthesis types

Material combination	*0.1–1.0 μm*	*1.0–10 μm*	*10–100 μm*
Zirconia-on-UHMWPE	1	0.17	0.04
Metal-on-metal	ND	–	–
Alumina-on-alumina (std.)	ND	–	–
Alumina-on-alumina (μsep)	0.19	–	–

ND, not determined; std., standard simulation conditions; μsep, micro-separation simulation conditions.

Table 2.3 Volumetric concentration *C*(*r*) of particles in each size range for each prosthesis type

Material combination	*0.1–1.0 μm*	*1.0–10 μm*	*10–100 μm*
Zirconia-on-UHMWPE	0.53	0.2	0.27
Metal-on-metal	1.0	–	–
Alumina-on-alumina (std.)	1.0	–	–
Alumina-on-alumina (μsep)	1.0	–	–

std., standard simulation conditions; μsep, micro-separation simulation conditions.

The index of specific biological activity (SBA) is shown in Table 2.4 for UHMWPE and alumina ceramic-on-ceramic tested under micro-separation simulation conditions. The SBA index of the alumina–ceramic particles was approximately one third that of the UHMWPE particles. The FBA indices for the zirconia-on-UHMWPE and alumina ceramic-on-ceramic prostheses are shown in Table 2.4. The alumina ceramic-on-ceramic prostheses produced an FBA value which was one fiftieth of that for zirconia-on-UHMWPE, which reflected the differences in volumetric wear rate and the reduced biological activity of the alumina–ceramic particles.

Table 2.4 SBA, volumetric wear, and FBA for wear particles generated by the different prosthesis types

Material combination	*SBA index*	*Volumetric wear rate ($mm^3/10^6$ cycles)*	*FBA index*
Zirconia-on-UHMWPE	0.57	31	18
Metal-on-metal	ND	1.6	ND
Alumina-on-alumina (std.)	ND	0.1	ND
Alumina-on-alumina (μsep)	0.19	1.84	0.35

ND, not determined; std., standard simulation conditions; μsep, micro-separation simulation conditions.

2.5 Discussion

This investigation of the wear of three different prostheses under clinically relevant conditions in the same simulator has demonstrated substantial differences in volumetric wear. The *in vitro* wear rates for the zirconia-on-UHMWPE and metal-on-metal couples are in agreement with clinical studies **(10)** and the UHMWPE and metal wear particles were similar to the wear debris isolated from retrieved tissues **(9, 22)**. The alumina–alumina wear rate generated under standard simulation conditions was one tenth to one fiftieth of that reported in some clinical retrieval studies, and the severe wear patterns observed *in vivo* **(39)** were not reproduced under standard simulation conditions. No change in surface roughness was detected by contacting profilometry, and only minimum damage was detected when the prostheses were examined using an interferometer. Ceramic wear particles as large as 7 μm have been identified *in vivo* **(46, 47)**, whereas the ceramic particles generated *in vitro* from the HIPed alumina material under standard simulation conditions were closer to 10 nm. These nanometre-sized wear particles were thought to be produced as a result of surface relief polishing of the alumina–ceramic. The introduction of micro-separation motion into the *in vitro* simulations reproduced the higher clinical wear rates and the stripe wear pattern on the femoral components. The wear rates increased from approximately 0.1 ±0.05 mm^3 per million cycles under standard simulation conditions to 1.84 ±0.3 mm^3 per million cycles under micro-separation simulation conditions. Rim contact was produced on heel strike along with elevated stress levels, which were consistent with *in vivo* conditions. This led to a wear stripe being produced on the femoral heads, which was comparable with the pattern observed on retrieved components. Surface roughness of the alumina–ceramic femoral heads increased after micro-separation testing to values comparable with retrieved components, indicating that wear mechanisms similar to those that occur *in vivo* were produced in the micro-separation simulation. In addition, under micro-separation simulation conditions, a bimodal distribution of particle sizes was observed. This bimodal distribution has been described recently in a series of retrieved Mittelmeier alumina ceramic-on-ceramic prostheses. Nanometre-sized (4–100 nm) particles were produced under micro-separation simulation conditions, together with larger micrometre-sized (0.1–3 μm) wear particles. The larger particles were thought to be produced from within the wear stripe by transgranular fracture of the alumina–ceramic material due to the elevated stress levels associated with the rim contact and relocation of the femoral head into the cup.

The biological effects of UHMWPE wear debris have been well documented **(2–6)**, and although the use of zirconia femoral heads produced lower wear volumes of UHMWPE than metal femoral heads, both *in vitro* (31 mm^3/million cycles compared to 35–45 mm^3/million cycles) **(58)** and clinically **(10)**, the volumetric particle load remains considerable. The majority of the UHMWPE wear debris isolated in this study was shown to be in the biologically active size range, with 73 per cent of particles (by mass) in the 0.1–10 μm size range. Previous studies have shown that particles in the 0.2–10 μm size range were biologically active, and stimulated macrophages to produce high levels of the pro-inflammatory cytokine TNF-α **(67)**.

The wear particles generated under standard simulation conditions from the MOM and COC articulations in this study were in the nanometre size range. Metal particles in the nanometre size range may produce necrosis of the tissues if sufficient volume is generated and accumulated in the periprosthetic tissues **(66)**. Clinical studies indicate that this is likely to be associated with volumetric wear rates greater than the 1 mm^3/million cycles recorded in this study. The biological effect of nanometre-sized alumina–ceramic particles is as yet poorly understood. However, Hatton *et al.* **(48)** showed that particles approximately 0.5 μm in size stimulated the production of TNF-α from peripheral blood mononuclear cells, albeit at a reduced level compared to that observed with UHMWPE particles of the same size. The present study has also shown that alumina particles produced under micro-separation simulation conditions demonstrated a five-fold lower biological activity index compared to UHMWPE particles. Determination of the FBA of the wear particles from the different materials under clinically relevant simulation conditions confirmed that the UHMWPE wear particles were the most biologically active with a three-fold higher specific biological activity compared to the alumina ceramic-on-ceramic particles generated under micro-separation simulation conditions. In addition, as the FBA index takes into account the wear volume of the materials, the FBA index for the zirconia-on-UHMWPE was some 50 times that of the alumina ceramic-on-ceramic wear particles generated under micro-separation conditions. As the wear volumes produced in ceramic-on-ceramic prostheses can be as much as 1000 times lower than polyethylene wear, the volume of ceramic particles *in vivo* may not reach sufficiently high levels to elicit an inflammatory response. Hence the incidence of osteolysis and loosening of ceramic implants may be considerably reduced. These studies indicate that the significantly lower wear volumes from the alumina ceramic-on-ceramic articulations confer a significant advantage over the more traditional articulations, which utilize UHMWPE as a bearing surface.

This work has revealed significant differences in the wear volumes, size distribution, and FBA of wear particles generated from the different prosthesis materials under clinically relevant conditions in *in vitro* wear simulators.

Acknowledgements

The work reported in this paper was performed in independent studies supported by the EPSRC, the ARC, the MRC, Depuy International, a Johnson and Johnson Company, and Stryker International Research and Development.

References

(1) **Malchau, H.** and **Herberts, P.** Prognosis of total hip replacement: surgical and cementing technique in THR: a revision study of 134 056 primary operations. In *Proceedings of the 63rd American Academy of Orthopaedic Surgeons*, Atlanta, 1996.

(2) **Campbell, P., Doorn, P., Dorey, F.,** and **Amstutz, H. C.** Wear and morphology of ultra-high molecular weight polyethylene wear particles from total hip replacements. *Proc. Instn. Mech. Engrs.*, 1996, **210H**, 167–74.

(3) **Goodman, S., Aspenberg, P., Song, Y., Knoblich, G., Huie, P., Regula, D.,** and **Lidgren, L.** Tissue ingrowth and differentiation in the bone-harvest chamber in the presence of cobalt chromium alloy and high density polyethylene particles. *J. Bone Jt Surg.*, 1995, **77-A**, 1025–1035.

(4) **Howie, D. W., Vernon-Roberts, B., Oakshott, R.,** and **Manthey, B.** A rat model of resorption of bone at the cement-bone interface in the presence of polyethylene wear particles. *J. Bone Jt Surg.*, 1988, **70-A**, 257–263.

(5) **Willert, H-G.** and **Semlitsch, M.** Reactions of the articular capsule to wear products of artificial joint prostheses. *J. Biomed. Mater. Res.*, 1977, **11**, 157–164.

(6) **Schmalzried, T. P., Jasty, M.,** and **Harris, W. H.** Periprosthetic bone loss in total hip arthroplasty: polyethylene wear debris and the concept of the effective joint space. *J. Bone Jt Surg.*, 1992, **74-A**, 849–863.

(7) **Kobayashi, A., Kadoya, Y., Bonfield, W., Revell, P. A., Yamac, T., Scott, G., Freeman, M. A. R., Ohashi, H.,** and **Yamano, Y.** Quantitative analysis of polyethylene wear particles in osteolytic regions around failed total joint prostheses. *Proceedings of the 43rd Orthopaedic Research Society*, San Francisco, 1997, pp. 68.

(8) **Hailey, J. L., Ingham, E., Stone, M. H., Wroblewski, B. M.,** and **Fisher J.** Ultra-high molecular weight polyethylene wear debris generated *in vivo* and in laboratory tests; the influence of counterface roughness. *Proc. Instn. Mech. Engrs.*, 1996, **210**, 3–10.

(9) **Tipper, J. L., Ingham, E., Hailey, J. L., Besong, A. A., Wroblewski, B. M., Stone, M. H.,** and **Fisher, J.** Quantitative analysis of polyethylene wear debris, wear rate and head damage in retrieved Charnley hip prostheses. *J. Mat Sci: Mats Med.*, 2000, **11**, 117–124.

(10) **Semlitsch, M.** and **Willert, H. G.** Clinical wear behaviour of ultra-high molecular weight polyethylene cups paired with metal and ceramic ball heads in comparison to metal-on-metal pairings of hip joint replacements. *Proc. Instn. Mech. Engrs.*, 1997, **211H**, 73–88.

(11) **Minakawa, H., Ingham, E., Tipper, J. L., Stone, M. H., Wroblewski, B. M.,** and **Fisher, J.** Why do ceramic femoral heads produce lower polyethylene wear in artificial joints? *Proc. Japan. Society Mech. Engrs.*, 1997, **205**, 331–334.

(12) **Jacobsson, S-A., Djerf, K.,** and **Wahlström, O.** 20 year results of McKee-Farrar versus Charnley Prostheses. *Clin. Orthop.*, 1996, **329**, S60–S68.

(13) **McKellop, H., Campbell, P., Park, S. H., Schmalzried, T. P., Grigoris, P., Amstutz, H. C.,** and **Sarmiento, A.** The origin of submicron polyethylene wear debris in total hip arthroplasty. *Clin. Orthop.*, 1995, **311**, 3–20.

(14) **McKellop, H., Park, S. H., Chiesa, R., Doorn, P., Lu, B., Normand, P., Grigoris, P.,** and **Amstutz, H. C.** *In vivo* wear of 3 types of metal on metal hip prostheses during 2 decades of use. *Clin. Orthop.*, 1996, **329**, S128–S140.

(15) **Semlitsch, M., Streicher, R. M.,** and **Weber, H.** Wear behaviour of cast CoCrMo cups and balls in long-term implanted total hip prostheses. *Orthopäde*, 1989, **18**, 377–381.

(16) **Clarke, I. C., Anissian, L., Stark, A., Gustafson, A., Good, V., Williams, P., Downs, B.,** and **Yu, L.** Comparisons of M-M and M-PE hip systems at 10 million cycles in hip simulator study. In *Metasul – A Metal on Metal Bearing* (Eds Rieker, C., Windler, M., and Wyss, U.), 1999, pp. 93–109 (Hans Huber, Bern).

(17) **Delaunay, C.** METASUL bearings in primary total hip arthroplasty: French experience. In *Metasul – A Metal on Metal Bearing* (Eds Rieker, C., Windler, M., and Wyss, U.), 1999, pp. 181–199 (Hans Huber, Bern).

(18) **Dörig, M. F., Odstreilik, E., Jovanovic, M.,** and **Kratter, R.** Uncemented alloclastic METASUL total hip arthroplasty: Early results after 2–6 years. In *Metasul – A Metal on Metal Bearing* (Eds Rieker, C., Windler, M., and Wyss, U.), 1999, pp. 157–170 (Hans Huber, Bern).

(19) **Dorr, L. D., Dubois, B.,** and **Wan, Z.** METASUL metal-on-metal articulation: Five year results. In *Metasul – A Metal on Metal Bearing* (Eds Rieker, C., Windler, M., and Wyss, U.), 1999, pp. 191–196 (Hans Huber, Bern).

(20) **Seiber, H. P., Rieker, C. B.,** and **Kottig, P.** Analysis of 118 second generation metal on metal retrieved hip implants. *J. Bone Jt Surg.*, 1998, **80-B**, 46–50.

(21) **Wagner, H.** and **Wagner, M.** German clinical results with METASUL bearings. In *Metasul – A Metal on Metal Bearing* (Eds Rieker, C., Windler, M., and Wyss, U.), 1999, pp. 171–180 (Hans Huber, Bern).

(22) **Doorn, P., Campbell, P., Worral, J., Benya, P., McKellop, H.,** and **Amstutz, H. C.** Metal wear particle characterisation from metal on metal total hip replacements: Transmission electron microscopy study of periprosthetic tissues and isolated particles. *J. Biomed. Mats. Res.*, 1998, **42**, 103–111.

(23) **Lee, J. M., Salvati, E. A., Betts, F., DiCarlo, E. F., Doty, S. B.,** and **Bullough, P. G.** Size of metallic and polyethylene debris particles in failed cemented total hip replacements. *J. Bone Jt Surg.*, 1992, **74-B**, 380–384.

(24) **Soh, E., Blunn, G. W., Wait, M. E.,** and **Walker, P. S.** Size and shape of metal particles from metal-on-metal total hip replacements. In *Proceedings of the 42nd Orthopaedic Research Society*, Atlanta, Georgia, 1996, pp. 462.

(25) **Case, C. P., Langkamer, V. G., James, C., Palmer, M. R., Kemp, A. J., Heap, P. F.,** and **Solomom, L.** Widespread dissemination of metal debris from implants. *J. Bone Jt Surg.*, 1994, **76-B**, 701–712.

(26) **Langkamer, V. G., Case, C. P., Heap, P., Taylor, A., Collins, C., Pearse, M.,** and **Solomom, L.** Systemic distribution of wear debris after hip replacement. *J. Bone Jt Surg.*, 1992, **74-B**, 831–839.

(27) **Shea, K. G., Lundeen, G. A., Bloebaum, R. D .,** and **Bachus, K. N.** Lymphoreticular dissemination of metal particulates in patients with primary joint replacements. In *Proceedings of the 42nd Orthopaedic Research Society*, Atlanta, Georgia, 1996, pp. 502.

(28) **Urban, R. M., Jacobs, J. J., Gavrilovic, J., Tomlinson, M. J., Black, J., Turner, T. M.,** and **Galante, J. O.** Dissemination of metal-alloy particles to the liver and spleen of patients with total hip or knee replacement prostheses. In *Proceedings of the 5th World Biomaterials Congress*, Toronto, Canada, 1996, pp. 660.

(29) **Hallab, N., Merritt, K.,** and **Jacobs, J. J.** Metal sensitivity in patients with orthopaedic implants. *J. Bone Jt Surg.*, 2001, **83-A**, 428–436.

(30) **Urban, R. M., Jacobs, J. J., Tomlinson, M. J., Gavrilovic, J., Black, J.,** and **Peoc'h, M.** Dissemination of wear particles to the liver, spleen and abdominal lymph nodes of patients with hip or knee replacement. *J. Bone Jt Surg.*, 2000, **82-A**, 457–477.

(31) **Beaulé, P. E., Campbell, P., Mirra, J., Hooper, J. C.,** and **Schmalzried, T. P.** Osteolysis in a cementless second generation metal-on-metal hip replacement. *Clin. Orthop.*, 2001, **386**, 159–165.
(32) **Schmalzried, T. P., Szuszczewick, E., Peterson, T. D.,** and **Amstutz, H. C.** Eliminating polyethylene will not put an end to osteolysis. *Orthopaedics (International Edition)*, 1999, **5**, 308–310.
(33) **Doorn, P. F., Mirra, J. M., Campbell, P. A.,** and **Amstutz, H. C.** Metal versus polyethylene wear particles in total hip replacements: A review. *Clin. Orthop.*, 1996, **329**, S187–S205.
(34) **Allen, M. J., Myer, B. J., Millet, P. J.,** and **Rushton, N.** The effects of particulate cobalt, chromium and cobalt-chromium alloy on human osteoblast-like cells *in vitro*. *J. Bone Jt Surg.*, 1997, **79-B**, 475–482.
(35) **Bendall, S. P., Radfar, A. J., Frondoza, C., Jinnah, R. H.,** and **Hungerford, D. S.** Metallic wear debris from periprosthetic tissue of failed arthroplasty induces TNF-α and IL-1α release from synoviocytes. In *Proceedings of the 5th World Biomaterials Congress*, Toronto, Canada, 1996, pp. 546.
(36) **Luchetti, W. T., Gonzales, J. B.,** and **Horowitz, S. M.** Osteoblast and macrophage reponses to cobalt chrome and titanium particles. In *Proceedings of the 5th World Biomaterials Congress*, Toronto, Canada, 1996, pp. 949.
(37) **Maloney, W. J., Smith, R. L., Castro, F.,** and **Schurman, D.** Fibroblast response to metallic debris *in vitro*. *J. Bone Jt Surg.*, 1993, **75-A**, 835–844.
(38) **Germain, M. A., Matthews, J. B., Stone, M. H., Fisher, J.,** and **Ingham, E.** The effect of clinically relevant cobalt chrome particles on the viability of human peripheral blood mononuclear cells and fibroblasts *in vitro*. In *Proceedings of the European Society for Biomaterials*, London, 2001, pp. T76.
(39) **Nevelos, J. E., Ingham, E., Doyle, C., Fisher, J.,** and **Nevelos, A. B.** Analysis of retrieved alumina ceramic components from Mittelmeier total hip prostheses. *Biomaterials*, 1999, **20**, 1833–1840.
(40) **Taylor, S. K., Serekian, P.,** and **Manley, M.** Wear performance of a contemporary alumina:alumina bearing couple under hip joint simulation. In *Proceedings of the 44th Orthopaedic Research Society*, New Orleans, Louisiana, 1998, pp. 51.
(41) **Oonishi, H., Nishida, M., Kawanabe, K., Yamamoto, K., Downs, B., Sorensen, K., Good, V., Braham, A.,** and **Clarke, I. C.** *In vitro* wear of AL2O3/Al2O3 implant combination with over 10 million cycles duration. In *Proceedings of the 45th Orthopaedic Research Society*, Anaheim, California, 1999, pp. 50.
(42) **Refior, H. J., Plitz, W.,** and **Walter, A.** *Ex vivo* and *in vitro* analysis of the alumina alumina bearing system for hip joint prostheses. In *Proceedings of the 10th International Symposium on Ceramics in Medicine*, 1997, **10**, 127–130.
(43) **Nevelos, J. E., Ingham, E., Doyle, C., Nevelos, A. B.,** and **Fisher, J.** The influence of acetabular cup angle on the wear of 'BIOLOX Forte' alumina ceramic bearing couples in a hip joint simulator. *J. Mat. Sci: Mats. Med.*, 2001, **12**, 141–144.
(44) **Nevelos, J., Ingham, E., Doyle, C., Striecher, R., Nevelos, A., Walter, W.,** and **Fisher, J.** Microseparation of the centres of alumina-alumina artificial hip joints during simulator testing procedures produces clinically relevant wear rates and patterns. *J. Arthroplasty*, 2000, **15**, 793–795.
(45) **Mallory, T. H., Dennis, D. A., Komistek, R. D., Northcut, E. J., Lombardi, A. V.,** and **Herrington, S. M.** Do total hip arthroplasties piston during leg length manoeuvres and Gait? An *in vitro* determination of total hip arthroplasty separation during

abduction/adduction leg lift and gait. *American Academy of Orthopaedic Surgeons*, Los Angeles, 1999, scientific exhibit 66.

(46) **Hatton, A., Ingham, E., Nevelos, J., Fisher, J.,** and **Nevelos, A.** Histological analysis of tissue from revised uncemented ceramic-on-ceramic total hip arthroplasties. In *Proceedings of the 6th World Biomaterials Congress*, Hawaii, 2000, pp. 1188.

(47) **Yoon, T. R., Rowe, S. M., Jung, S. T., Seon, K. J.,** and **Maloney, W. J.** Osteolysis in association with a total hip arthroplasty with ceramic bearing surfaces. *J. Bone Jt Surg.*, 1998, **80-A**, 1459–1468.

(48) **Hatton, A., Ingham, E., Matthews, J. B.,** and **Fisher, J.** Cytokine release by human peripheral blood macrophages after stimulation with alumina ceramic particles *in vitro* – a comparison with UHMWPE. In *Proceedings of the 6th World Biomaterials Congress*, Hawaii, 2000, pp. 1186.

(49) **Wang, A. Stark, C.,** and **Dumbleton, J. H.** Mechanistic and morphological origins of ultra-high molecular weight polyethylene wear debris in total joint replacement prostheses. *Proc. Instn. Mech. Engrs.*, 1996, **210H**, 141–155.

(50) **Bragdon, C. R., O'Connor, D. O., Lowenstein, J. D., Jasty, M.,** and **Syniuta, W. D.** The importance of multidirectional motion on the wear of polyethylene. *Proc. Instn. Mech. Engrs.*, 1996, **210H**, 157–165.

(51) **Wang, A., Sun, D. C., Yau, S-S., Edwards, B., Sokol, M., Essner, A., Polineni, V. K., Stark, C.,** and **Dumbleton, J. H.** Orientation softening in the deformation and wear of ultra-high molecular weight polyethylene. *Wear*, 1997, **203–204**, 230–241.

(52) **McKellop, H. A.** and **Röstund, T. V.** The wear behaviour of ion-implanted Ti-6Al-4V against UHMW polyethylene. *J. Biomed. Mater. Res.*, 1990, **24**, 1413–1425.

(53) **Bigsby, R. J. A., Hardaker, C. S.,** and **Fisher, J.** Wear of ultra-high molecular weight polyethylene in a physiological hip joint simulator in the anatomical position using bovine serum as a lubricant. *Proc. Instn. Mech. Engrs.*, 1997, **211H**, 265–270.

(54) **Besong, A. A., Bigsby, R. J. A., Barbour, P. S. M.,** and **Fisher, J.** Effect of head size and loading regime on the wear of UHMWPE acetabular cups in a hip simulator. In *Proceedings of the World Tribology Congress*, London, 1997, pp. 732.

(55) **Saikko, V. O.** A three-axis hip joint simulator for wear and friction studies on total hip prostheses. *Proc. Instn. Mech. Engrs.*, 1996, **210H**, 175–186.

(56) **Derbyshire, B., Fisher, J., Dowson, D., Hardaker, C. S.,** and **Brummitt, K.** Comparative study of the wear of UHMWPE with zirconia ceramic and stainless steel femoral heads in artificial hip joints. *Med. Engng Phys.*, 1994, **16**, 229–236.

(57) **Paul, J. P.** Forces transmitted by joints in the human body. *Proc. Instn. Mech. Engrs.*, 1967, **23**, 8–15.

(58) **Barbour, P. S. M., Stone, M. H.,** and **Fisher, J.** A hip joint simulator study using simplified loading and motion cycles generating physiological wear paths and rates. *Proc. Instn. Mech. Engrs.*, 1999, **213H**, 455–467.

(59) **Medley, J. B., Chan, F. W., Krygier, J. J.,** and **Bobyn, J. D.** Comparisons of alloys and designs in a hip simulator study. *Clin. Orthop.*, 1996, **329**, S148–S159.

(60) **McKellop, H., Lu, B.,** and **Wiser, H.** The effect of specimen orientation and lubricant concentration on the wear of metal/metal hip implants in a wear simulator. In *Proceedings of the 45th Orthopaedic Research Society*, Anaheim, California, 1999, pp. 849.

(61) **Derbyshire, B., Hardaker, C. S., Fisher, J., Dowson, D.,** and **Brummitt, K.** Assessment of the change in volume of acetabular cups using a co-ordinate measuring machine. *Proc. Instn. Mech. Engrs*, 1994, **208H**, 151–158.

(62) **Besong, A. A., Tipper, J. L., Ingham, E., Stone, M. H., Wroblewski, B. M.**, and **Fisher, J.** Quantitative comparison of wear debris that has and has not been sterilised by gamma irradiation. *J. Bone Jt Surg.*, 1998, **80-B**, 340–344.

(63) **Fisher, J., Bell, J., Barbour, P. S. M., Tipper, J. L., Matthews, J. B., Besong, A. A., Stone, M. H.**, and **Ingham, E.** A novel method for the prediction of functional biological activity of polyethylene wear debris. *Proc. Instn. Mech. Engrs.*, 2001, **215H**, 127–132.

(64) **Matthews, J. B., Besong, A. A., Green, T. R., Stone, M. H., Wroblewski, B. M., Fisher, J.**, and **Ingham, E.** Evaluation of the response of primary human peripheral blood mononuclear phagocytes to challenge with *in vitro* generated clinically relevant UHMWPE particles of known size and dose. *J. Biomed. Mater. Res.*, 2000, **52**, 296–307.

(65) **Green, T. R., Fisher, J., Matthews, J. B., Stone, M. H.**, and **Ingham, E.** Effect of size and dose on bone resorption activity of macrophages by *in vitro* clinically relevant ultra high molecular weight polyethylene particles. *J. Biomed. Mater. Res.*, 2000, **53**, 490–497.

(66) **Schwarz, E. M., Lu, A. P., Goater, J., Benz, E. B., Kollias, G., Rosier, R. N., Puzas, J. E.**, and **O'Keefe, R. J.** Tumour necrosis factor-α/nuclear transcription factor-κB signalling in periprosthetic osteolysis. *J. Orthop. Res.*, 2000, **18**, 472–480.

(67) **Green, T. R., Fisher, J., Stone, M. H., Wroblewski, B. M.**, and **Ingham, E.** Polyethylene particles of a 'critical size' are necessary for the induction of cytokines by macrophages *in vitro*. *Biomaterials*, 1998, **19**, 2297–2302.

J L Tipper, J B Matthews, and **E Ingham**
Medical and Biological Engineering, Division of Microbiology, University of Leeds, UK
T D Stewart and **J Fisher**
Medical and Biological Engineering, School of Mechanical Engineering, University of Leeds, UK
M H Stone
Department of Orthopaedic Surgery, Leeds General Infirmary, UK

3

The Influence of Component Geometry on the Measurement of Wear

J A Williams and **J J Kauzlarich**

Abstract

The wear performance of tribological material pairs is commonly assessed by experimental investigations which make use of specimen geometries which differ from those of the components to be used in service. The information so generated is conventionally interpreted in terms of a linear relation between wear volume, applied load, and sliding distance in accord with the Archard wear equation. An appropriate material parameter is thus the so-called dimensional wear rate usually measured in $mm^3\ N^{-1}\ m^{-1}$. However, there are many practical situations not least in medical prostheses in which, as components wear, the area of apparent contact changes so that although the Archard relation may still be applicable at the micro-scale, the macroscopic wear dimension, or the total wear volume, may be other than a linear function of sliding distance or load. In this contribution, we consider how to relate data acquired in one geometric arrangement to dimensional and volumetric wear in another.

Notation

B	bearing or chord length
b	radius ratio, R/r
K_w	dimensional wear constant
L	sliding distance
N	number of revolutions
P	nominal bearing pressure
R	larger sphere radius
r	smaller sphere radius
V	volumetric wear
W	load
Δ	dimensional wear
$\alpha, \beta, \gamma, \varepsilon$	surface contact angles

3.1 Introduction

Wear is a commonplace phenomenon. In the field of machine design and operation, the 'running-in', or 'wearing-in', of a rubbing machine element is often beneficial whereas premature wear-out of the same element is highly undesirable. In order to accommodate this behaviour engineering designers need access to predictive governing equations which take account of practical material combinations, realistic component geometries, and appropriate operating conditions.

There has been controversy concerning wear theory for over a century and it is improbable that a single governing equation will be established to cover all eventualities. However, it has been demonstrated that for a wide range of conditions, both 'adhesive' and 'abrasive', the wear volume V, load W, and sliding distance L are related by an equation of the form

$$V = \mathrm{K_w}\, WL \tag{3.1}$$

where $\mathrm{K_w}$ is termed the dimensional wear coefficient and is conventionally quoted in units of $\mathrm{mm^3\ N^{-1}\ m^{-1}}$. Its numerical value is characteristic of the material pair used as the wearing couple and the imposed environmental conditions. An equation of this form was postulated by Preston **(1)** in relation to the abrasive polishing of glass and is consequently known as the Preston equation to those involved with this and similar technologies. It was likewise proposed by Archard in relation to adhesive wear **(2, 3)** and extended by Rabinowicz to more general cases of abrasive wear **(4)** and is often known as the Archard equation. The numerical value of the 'constant' $\mathrm{K_w}$ can vary enormously; situations of very mild wear generating values less than $10^{-9}\ \mathrm{mm^3\ N^{-1}\ m^{-1}}$ while values of 10^{-4} or more would generally be considered unacceptably severe for most tribological situations.

Although some progress has been made in relating the value of $\mathrm{K_w}$ to more fundamental or intrinsic material properties and relevant operating conditions **(5)** the most significant sources of guidance to practical values are experimental investigations. Most of these are carried out using a simple pin-on-disc arrangement, as illustrated in Fig. 3.1(a), where the prismatic (usually cylindrical) pin is a specimen of the wearing material and the disc represents the more wear resistant counterface. Wear volume is assessed either by the change in the length of the pin or by its loss in mass or volume, the load W is usually applied as a dead weight and the length of the sliding path is simply related to the number of revolutions of the disc. Providing the wearing surface remains parallel to the abrading disc this simple arrangement has the advantage that the apparent contact area and thus the nominal pressure on the wearing pin remains constant during the course of the test. On the basis of equation (3.1), dividing each side by the cube of the pin radius

$$\frac{V}{r^3} = \pi \times \mathrm{K_w} \times \frac{W}{\pi r^2} \times \frac{L}{r} \tag{3.2}$$

so that if we define a 'nominal pressure' P as the load divided by the 'foot-print' of the contact area and normalize the sliding distance L by the pin radius r to give $L/r = N$ we can write

$$\frac{V}{r^3} = \pi \mathrm{K_w}\, PN \tag{3.3}$$

The group K_wPN can be thought of as a 'service parameter'; high loads, large sliding distances, or material pairs prone to wear (i.e. with a high value of K_w) all increase its value. However, in order to ease alignment problems during setting-up, the pin is often given a spherical tip which gradually wears away; during this 'running-in' process the area of the contact is growing while the load remains the same so that even if the Archard law is obeyed on the very local scale the overall dimensional loss will no longer grow linearly with sliding distance. There are many other situations, both of potential test geometries and practical devices in the field, where the apparent contact area changes with wear and/or sliding distance. Three examples are illustrated in Fig. 3.1(b)–(d). Figure 3.1(b) represents a crossed cylinder test geometry in which the upper cylinder rotates. This can either be of the harder or more aggressive material (so concentrating the wear on the softer lower member at a single wear scar), or it can be the softer material itself so that the test procedure generates a circumferential wear track. Figure 3.1(c) illustrates a simple journal bearing arrangement in which the rotating shaft or journal is gradually producing an axial groove in the softer bearing sleeve and Fig. 3.1(d) represents a spherical bearing in which a hard sphere rotates in a spherical housing or cup. The geometry of the latter two examples are analogous to simplified orthopaedic prostheses.

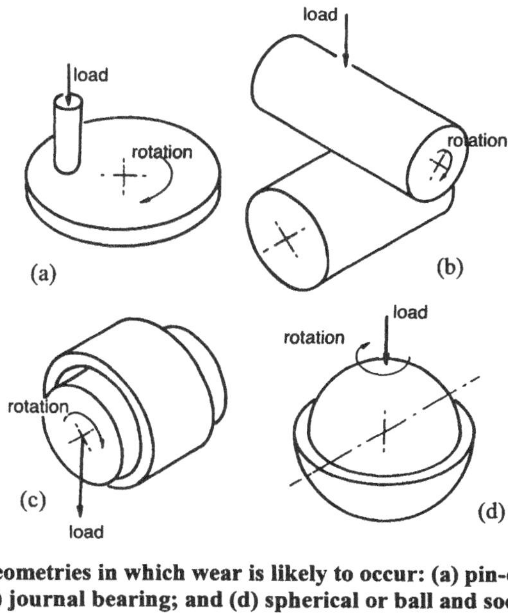

Fig. 3.1 Contact geometries in which wear is likely to occur: (a) pin-on-disc; (b) crossed cylinder; (c) journal bearing; and (d) spherical or ball and socket bearing

In each case, although at the local scale the wear behaviour of the softer material might be governed by a relationship between local loads and sliding distances of the form of equation (3.1) it is not immediately obvious that this linear relation will be exhibited by the contact as a whole. In addition, to the design engineer or end-user it is often the rate at which the dimensional tolerance of the contact grows (rather than the volumetric loss) that is of significance. It is this that dictates the rate at which the bearing loosens with use so generating a consequential loss of location accuracy in any device of which the wearing element is a part.

3.2 Spherical ended pin or pivot

3.2.1 Sliding contacts

Consider a spherically ended pin or slider of radius r carrying a normal load W sliding against a plane surface. Further, suppose that it is the sphere that wears and that at any point on the interface between the two materials the Archard wear law is obeyed with a constant dimensional wear coefficient of magnitude K_w.

Working in terms of the angle β_0 defined in Fig. 3.2

$$\frac{\Delta}{r} = 1 - \cos\beta_0 \tag{3.4}$$

and

$$\frac{V}{r^3} = \frac{\pi}{3}\left(2 - 3\cos\beta_0 + \cos^3\beta_0\right) \tag{3.5}$$

where V is the volume lost by wear from the sphere.

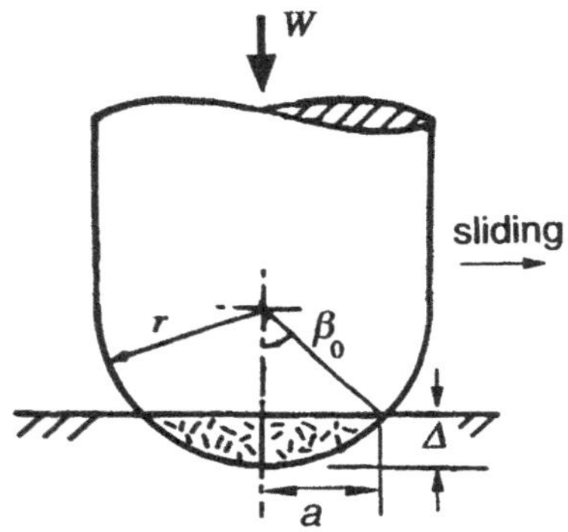

Fig. 3.2 A spherically (or cylindrically) ended pin of radius r carrying load W wearing against a flat counterface – the shaded area of depth Δ represents the volume V worn from the pin

Over the next increment of time suppose the volume lost from the sphere is $\mathrm{d}V$ while the distance slid by the contact is $\mathrm{d}L$, then equation (3.1) becomes

$$\mathrm{d}V = K_w W \mathrm{d}L$$

but

$$\mathrm{d}V = \mathrm{d}\Delta\, \pi a^2$$

where

$$a = r\sin\beta_0$$

see Fig. 3.2, and by differentiating equation (3.4)

$$\mathrm{d}\Delta = r\sin\beta_0\mathrm{d}\beta_0$$

thus

$$\mathrm{K_w}P\mathrm{d}N = \pi\sin^3\beta_0\mathrm{d}\beta_0$$

where P and N are defined as before.

But since

$$\int_0^{\beta_0}\sin^3\beta_0\mathrm{d}\beta_0 = \frac{1}{12}\left(2-3\cos\beta_0+\cos^3\beta_0\right)$$

it follows, from equation (3.5), that the normalized volumetric wear is related to the service parameter by the equation

$$\frac{V}{r^3} = \pi\mathrm{K_w}\,PN$$

just as is the case for a flat ended pin. The normalized dimensional wear rate Δ/r can be found by eliminating β_0 between equations. (3.1), (3.4), and (3.5) to give the expression

$$\left\{\frac{\Delta}{r}\right\}^2 \times \left\{1-\frac{\Delta}{r}\right\} = \mathrm{K_w}PN \tag{3.6}$$

In the initial stages of wear, when Δ/r and the angle β_0 are small, then this can be approximated by

$$\frac{\Delta}{r} \approx \sqrt{(\mathrm{K_w}PN)} \tag{3.7}$$

The validity of this approach can be tested by comparing the outcome both to direct experimental observation and to results computed by numerical simulation. In a recent publication Pödra and Andersson **(6)** have examined the initial rate of dimensional loss in a simple pin-on-disc test in which a sacrificial pin with an initial tip radius of 5 mm was slid under a constant normal load of either 21 N or 50 N against a harder steel substrate. This process was modelled by an incremental finite element analysis. Figure 3.3 shows a comparison of both their computed dimensional wear curves and their measured data points for the two load values with that generated by equation (3.7) above. The mean wear coefficient used in both the FEA simulation and the application of equation (3.7) was $\mathrm{K_w} = 1.33 \times 10^{-13}\ \mathrm{Pa^{-1}}$, i.e. $1.33 \times 10^{-4}\ \mathrm{mm^3\ N^{-1}\ m^{-1}}$.

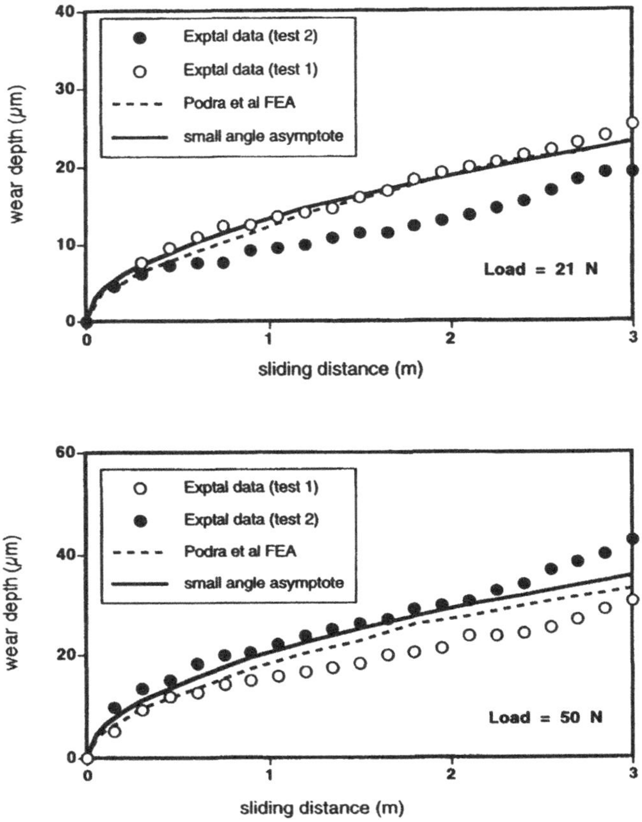

Fig. 3.3 Comparison of experimental data and finite element analysis [both from reference (6)] with simplified small angle asymptotes for wear of a spherically ended pin; (a) normal load of 21 N, and (b) normal load of 50 N – in both cases wear coefficient $K_w = 1.33 \times 10^{-4}$ mm^{-3} N^{-1} m^{-1}

3.2.2 Spherical pivot

If the pin *rotates* about its own axis instead of sliding, and if N is now the total number of revolutions completed by the pin, equations (3.1) and (3.7) are replaced by

$$\frac{V}{r^3} \approx 0.25 \times \left(3^4 \pi^7\right)^{1/3} \times \left(K_w P N\right)^{4/3} \tag{3.8}$$

$$\frac{\Delta}{r} \approx 0.5 \times (3\pi)^{2/3} \times \left(K_w P N\right)^{2/3} \tag{3.9}$$

These are identical to the corresponding equations, viz (3.10) and (3.13), derived by Kauzlarich *et al.* (7) for this geometry where it is the originally hemispherically ended shaft that is sacrificial.

3.2.3 Sliding cylindrical contact

In the case of a softer cylinder, of length *B*, sliding in a direction normal to its axis, the appropriate expressions for the initial dimensional and volumetric wear rates are, respectively

$$\frac{\Delta}{r} \approx 0.5 \times (9)^{1/3} \times (K_w PN)^{2/3} \tag{3.10}$$

and

$$\frac{V}{r^3} \approx 2 \times K_w PN\, V/Br^2$$

where

$$P = W/2Br \tag{3.11}$$

3.3 Other test geometries

Common to the geometries illustrated in Fig. 3.1(b), (c), and (d) is the fact that as wear progresses the area of contact increases; all can be analysed in an analogous fashion to that of a sliding wear pin, see reference **(8)**. As an example, consider Fig. 3.1(d) in which a loaded ball, radius *r*, is supported in a spherical housing or cup which has radius *R* equal to *br*. This situation is illustrated in Fig 3.4. The normal load is again *W* and *N* is now the number of revolutions of the sphere about, say, the axis indicated.

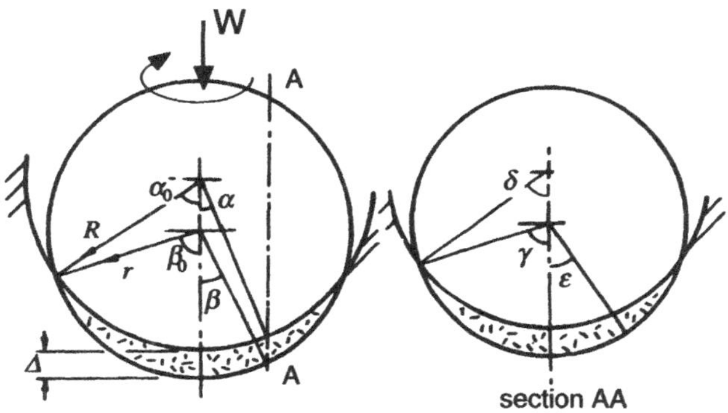

Fig. 3.4 Geometry of a wearing spherical bearing – the rotating sphere of radius *r* carries a uniform and stationary load *W* (dimension *Δ* represents the depth by which the sphere has penetrated the softer surrounding bearing cup which is of radius *R* = *br*)

The normalized dimensional wear is simply related to the angles α_0 and β_0

$$\frac{\Delta}{r} = (1-\cos\beta_0) - b(1-\cos\alpha_0) \quad \text{where } \alpha_0 = \arcsin[(\sin\beta_0)/b] \tag{3.12}$$

and the volumetric wear loss *V* is given by

$$\frac{V}{r^3} = \frac{\pi}{3}\left\{\left(2 - 3\cos\beta_0 + \cos^3\beta_0\right) - b^3\left(2 - 3\cos\alpha_0 + \cos^3\alpha_0\right)\right\} \tag{3.13}$$

The interfacial pressure between the sphere and the worn surface of the cup is not known *a priori* but at all times must be such that at all times both overall equilibrium of forces is satisfied and that at every point at the sliding interface Archard wear is taking place. On this basis it is possible to show **(8)** that

$$\mathrm{K_w}PN = \frac{2}{\pi^2}\int_0^{\beta_0} \mathrm{I}(\sin\beta_0 \tan\alpha_0 \cos\beta_0) d\beta_0 \tag{3.14}$$

where

$$\mathrm{I} = \int_0^{\beta_0}\int_0^{\gamma} \cos^2\varepsilon \cos^3\beta \; \mathrm{d}\varepsilon \; \mathrm{d}\beta$$

and

$$\cos\gamma = \cos\beta_0 / \cos\beta$$

When the angle β_0 is small, equations (3.12), (3.13), and (3.14) reduce to

$$\frac{\Delta}{r} \approx \sqrt{[\pi(1 - 1/b)]} \times \sqrt{(\mathrm{K_w}PN)} \tag{3.15}$$

and

$$\frac{V}{r^3} \approx \pi^2 \times \mathrm{K_w}PN \tag{3.16}$$

On the other hand, when β_0 approaches 90 degrees the situation is one in which the sphere ‘tunnels’ into the seat. The corresponding large angle asymptotes are

$$\frac{\Delta}{r} = 3\pi \times \mathrm{K_w}PN \tag{3.17}$$

and

$$\frac{V}{r^3} = 3\pi^2 \times \mathrm{K_w}PN \tag{3.18}$$

Note that both equations (3.16) and (3.18) suggest linear relationships between the volumetric loss and the service parameter $\mathrm{K_w}PN$ but that the leading coefficient changes by a factor three from initial- to steady-state conditions.

Figures 3.5 and 3.6 illustrate the match between these approximate solutions and the exact solutions represented by equations (3.12), (3.13), and (3.14). Values of b equal to 1.003, 1.02, 1.1, 2, 5, and 20 have been chosen. In the plot of Δ/r versus the service group $\mathrm{K_w}PN$ there is a clear transition from the initial region, where in this case the slope is one half, to a linear region at greater wearing distances. It can be noted that eliminating the group $\mathrm{K_w}PN$ between equations (3.17) and (3.18) (when β_0 is large) recovers the conventional tunnelling equation

$$\frac{V}{r^3} = \pi \times \frac{\Delta}{r} \tag{3.19}$$

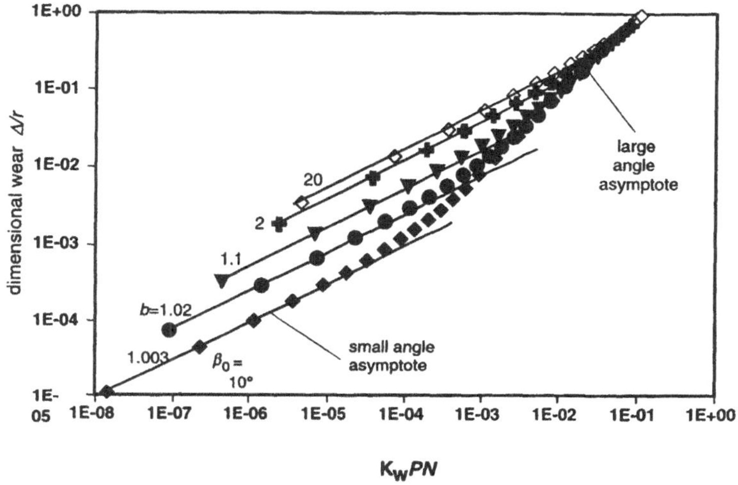

Fig. 3.5 Dimensional wear Δ/r as a function of the parameter K_wPN for spherical bearing geometry – data points computed from equations (3.12) and (3.14) for values of β_0 from 5 to 90 degrees at 5 degree intervals [solid lines are asymptotes, equations (3.15) and (3.17), referred to in the text]

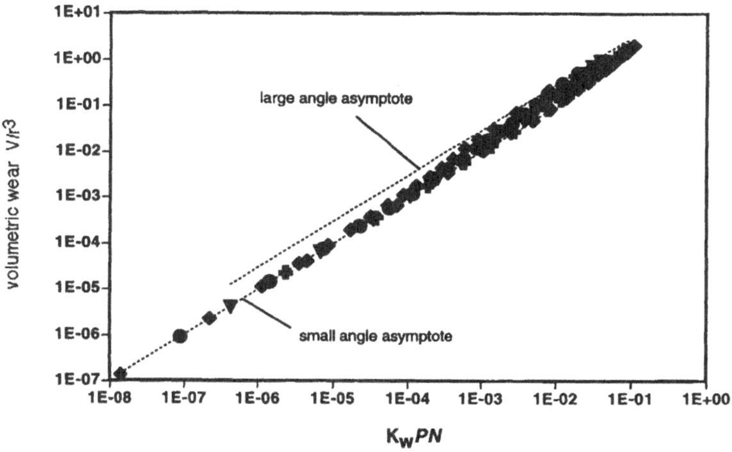

Fig. 3.6 Volumetric wear V/r^3 as a function of the parameter K_wPN for spherical bearing geometry – data points computed from equations (3.13) and (3.14) for values of β_0 from 5 to 90 degrees at 5 degree intervals [solid lines are asymptotes, equations (3.16) and (3.18), referred to in the text]

Dowson, Jobbins, and Seyed-Harraf **(9)** have presented both volumetric and dimensional wear data from tests on a hip prosthesis in which a steadily loaded alumina femoral head was reciprocated in an ultra-high, molecular-weight polythene (UHMWPE) acetabular cup. Figure 3.7 shows a plot of the penetration of two heads into the cups, i.e. the extent of dimensional wear as a function of the number of loading cycles during each of which the head moved through an angle of 55 degrees. Six data points are shown. The difference in radii between head and cup corresponded to a value of b = 1.02 and the load was such that the mean pressure P was 3.62 MPa. The solid line is a plot of equation (3.15) using these values together with a value of K_w equal to 4.58×10^{-7} mm^3 N^{-1} m^{-1}. The experimentally determined mean value is very close, being quoted as 4.49×10^{-7} mm^3 N^{-1} m^{-1}. Values of the angle β_0, established from equation (3.14), are indicated by the triangles on the computed curve of Fig. 3.7.

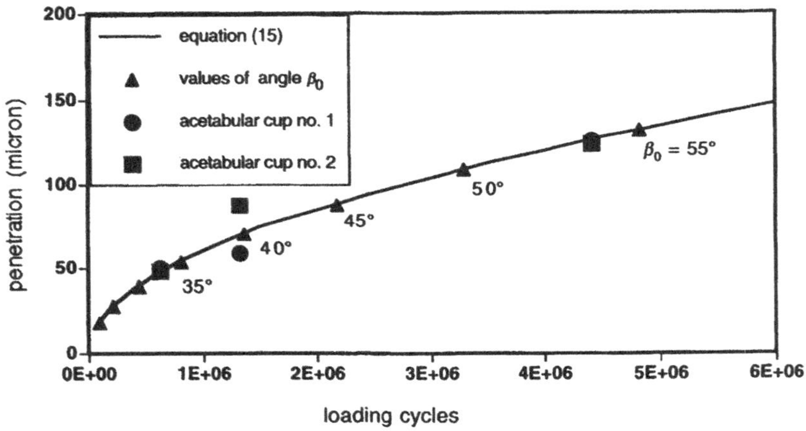

Fig. 3.7 Penetration of an alumina femoral head into UHMWPE acetabular cup [data points from reference (9)] curve computed from equation (3.15)

3.4 Conclusions

The resistance of a material to wear is often assessed using a test geometry which is different from those of real components which might be manufactured from it. In particular, wear tests are often carried out using a pin-on-disc arrangement, in which the test material is the sacrificial pin. In order to translate empirical data from such tests to field conditions involving sliding contacts, such as occur in spherical or other bearings, the resistance of the material to dry wear is conventionally expressed in units of volume lost per unit sliding distance per unit normal load. This is often known as the dimensional wear resistance K_w. This can be normalized by dividing by the value of the material hardness to give a non-dimensional wear resistance.

Even if every element at the loaded and wearing interface in the field application behaves locally in accordance with the Archard wear law, i.e. there is a linear relation between incremental wear volumes and local loads and sliding distances, it is not immediately obvious how the overall or global volumetric wear loss from the component will be related to the total applied load or global sliding history. This is because the interfacial pressure is not known *a priori* but will rather adjust itself as wear proceeds in such a way that both the demands of force equilibrium are satisfied and the overall wear geometry is consistent with the maintenance of geometric compatibility between both elements of the tribological pair.

We demonstrate here that for a spherically ended pin rubbing on a flat and for a spherical bearing, at any stage from initial contact to final steady-state conditions, the short-time volumetric wear loss increases linearly with both load and incremental sliding distance. However, in the case of spherical bearings the leading coefficient in this relation is not constant, so that total volume loss = f(sliding distance) × (K_w × load × sliding distance).

In addition, when wear is expressed in terms of dimensional loss, then in both these cases the initial rate of dimensional wear growth is dependent on the square root of the group (K_w × load × sliding distance). The assumption of linearity between wear and either load or sliding distance during this 'running-in' stage can lead to very significant errors in estimates of values of K_w.

In a further paper these relations are explored for a number of other wearing geometries **(8)** and these can be verified by appeal to a number of wear studies in the literature. We have not evaluated frictional torque or sliding resistance although these can be readily determined from a knowledge of the local interfacial stress distribution and geometry which form intrinsic elements of the analysis presented, following the methods suggested by Kauzlarich *et al.* **(7)**. Finally, we should add the proviso that this Chapter does not take into account any fundamental changes in wear mechanism that may occur during the life of the component due, for example, to the generation of transfer films on the counterface or the loss of material though some form of fatigue or delamination mechanism which requires the accumulation, with time, of subsurface damage.

Acknowledgement

The authors would like to express their appreciation for the comments and suggestions offered by Dr J A Greenwood and Professor K L Johnson.

References

(1) **Preston, F. W.** Theory and design of plate glass polishing machines. *J. Soc. Glass Tech.*, 1927, 11, 214–256.

(2) **Archard, J. F.** and **Hirst, W.** Wear of metals under unlubricated conditions. *Proc. Roy. Soc.*, 1956, A236, 3–55.

(3) **Archard, J. F.** Contact and rubbing of flat surfaces. *J. Applied Physics*, 1953, 24, 981–988.

(4) **Rabinowicz, E.** *Friction and Wear of Materials*, 1965, John Wiley, New York.

(5) **Williams, J. A.** Wear modelling: analytical, computational and mapping: a continuum mechanics approach. *Wear*, 1999, 225–229, 1–17.

(6) **Põdra, P.** and **Andersson, S.** Simulating sliding wear with finite element method. *Tribology International,* 1999, 32, 71–81.

(7) **Kauzlarich, J. J., Bhatia, K. G.,** and **Streitman, H. W.** Effect of wear on pivot thrust bearings. *Trans American Soc. Lubrication Engineers,* 1966, 9, 257–263. Correction: Fig. 4 is incorrect; replot equation 13, and correct data for run-in after 5.9×10^5 revolutions by 4.4 in^3.

(8) **Kauzlarich, J. J.** and **Williams, J. A.** Archard wear and component geometry. *Proc. Instn Mech. Engrs, J. Engng. Tribology,* 2001, 215, 387–403.

(9) **Dowson, D., Jobbins, B.,** and **Seyed-Harraf, A.** An evaluation of the penetration of ceramic femoral heads into polythene acatabular cups. *Wear,* 1993, 162–164, 880–889.

J A Williams
Engineering Department, Cambridge University, UK
J J Kauzlarich
Department of Mechanical Engineering, University of Virginia, Charlottesville, USA

4

A Tribological Study of Metal-on-metal Total Replacement Hip Joints

D Dowson, A A J Goldsmith, C M McNie, and S L Smith

Abstract

The resurgence of interest in hard-on-hard total replacement hip joints in recent years has promoted a number of studies on wear and lubrication in metal-on-metal implants. The wear of such implants is strongly influenced by joint geometry, particularly diameter, clearance and sphericity, materials of construction, and surface finish.

In this Chapter the results from a number of laboratory investigations carried out over several years on a ProSim multi-station hip simulator will be reviewed. The laboratory studies fall into two categories: investigations of the role of joint geometry upon wear and a search for lubricating films by means of a voltage-drop technique. The latter studies have been supplemented by simple analytical predictions of elasto-hydrodynamic film thickness for representative mean values of the speed, load, and viscosity encountered in the walking cycle.

The evidence gleaned from both the experimental and theoretical studies suggests that the severity of direct metal-to-metal interaction can be much relieved by effective lubrication of the joint during a substantial part of each loading cycle. Current understanding of the tribological characteristics of metal-on-metal joints will be reviewed.

The understanding achieved provides an opportunity for the optimization of design and manufacture of metal-on-metal implants through the application of tribological principles. The provision of maximum relief from the severity of wear in metal-on-metal joints by effective lubrication in simulated walking cycles, on well controlled laboratory simulators, is a necessary, but by no means sufficient, step towards optimization of implant performance. Investigations of the effect of frequent interruptions to the loading and motion cycles, which represent more fully daily experience, are required. Further studies of the role of material composition and structure upon wear, and consideration of the behaviour of wear debris in the bearing clearance, are also required.

Notation

c_d diametral clearance $[= 2\,(r_c - r_h)]$
d diameter of femoral head
h_{min} minimum film thickness
k wear factor
r_h radius of femoral head
r_c radius of acetabular cup
u entraining velocity $(u_h + u_c)/2$
u_c surface velocity of acetabular cup
u_h surface velocity of femoral head
w applied load
x sliding distance
E modulus of elasticity
E' effective elastic modulus $E' = 2 \Big/ \left[\dfrac{1 - v_h^2}{E_h} + \dfrac{1 - v_c^2}{E_c}\right]$
H_{min} dimensionless minimum film thickness (h_{min}/R)
P load
R effective radius of an equivalent sphere near a plane

$$\frac{1}{R} = \left[\frac{1}{r_h} - \frac{1}{r_c}\right] \quad or \quad R = (d/2)[(d/c_d) + 1] \approx (d^2/2c_d)$$

R_a arithmetic mean roughness
V volume of material removed by wear
v Poisson's ratio
η lubricant viscosity

4.1 Introduction

The hip-joint replacement field has been largely dominated by metal-on-polymer prostheses of the Charnley type for almost half a century **(1)**. However, concern for loosening, and the limitations imposed upon, implant life by osteolysis promoted by polyethylene wear debris has resulted in a search for alternative material combinations. The pioneering development initiated in the 1950s by McKee and Watson-Farrar **(2)** has attracted renewed interest in metal-on-metal total hip replacements in recent years. Some of these earlier designs of metal-on-metal implants survived for 20 or 30 years **(3–5)**, although the majority failed much earlier.

A growing body of evidence has suggested that for materials, such as polyethylene, there is a threshold volume of wear debris which distinguishes between adequate performance and loosening of THR components **(6–8)**. A reduction in the joint wear rate might therefore extend prosthetic life by delaying the onset of loosening. It is primarily for this reason that there has been a resurgence of interest **(1)** in hard-on-hard implants such as metal-on-metal and ceramic-on-ceramic. It is the former that is of interest here.

The performance of well-designed and manufactured metal-on-metal joints can be quite spectacular. Wear rates can be some two orders of magnitude lower than those of conventional metal-on-polyethylene joints **(5, 9)** of 22.225 mm diameter. However, polyethylene wear debris is generally much larger than metallic debris, the former having a size typically in the range 0.1–0.5 μm **(10, 11)** and the latter between about 0.015–0.025 μm **(12, 13)**. For similar volumes of polyethylene and metal debris, the number of metallic particles will thus be approximately two or three orders of magnitude greater than the number of polyethylene particles. This order of magnitude analysis suggests that the much reduced wear volumes found in metal-on-metal implants, compared to metal-on-polymer alternatives, will not necessarily lead to a reduction in the number of wear particles.

The biological response to both polyethylene and metallic wear particles thus assumes some importance. Studies of macrophage response to wear debris have indicated that differences in particle size **(14)**, material **(15)**, morphology **(16)**, and surface charge **(17)** can all elicit various adverse biological responses. The concept of functional biological activity in relation to wear debris in joint replacements has been developed in some detail in references **(18–20)**.

It nevertheless remains important to understand the factors controlling wear in different forms of implants. Some of the tribological studies of metal-on-metal joints reviewed here indicate directly for the first time an intriguing behaviour, which accords with wider experience of certain industrial bearings. It also indicates that the mode of lubrication in well-designed and carefully manufactured metal-on-metal joints can be quite different from the boundary lubrication mechanism that dominates the performance of metal-on-polymer and most other forms of implants in common use.

It has become evident that it is primarily the formation of protective lubricating films that reduces wear in such a spectacular way in metal-on-metal implants. The experimental evidence has been summarized in **(21)** and related to the well-established Stribeck curve originally introduced early in the 20th century **(22)** in studies of friction in steadily loaded journal bearings.

If the use of metal-on-metal hip joints is to become more widespread and successful, it is important that the tribological principles governing their operation are understood and applied to new designs.

4.2 Materials and methods

4.2.1 The hip-joint simulator

The laboratory studies were undertaken on a ten-station ProSim hip-joint simulator **(23)**. The components were anatomically mounted at 35 degrees to the horizontal with the resultant load vector displaced medially by approximately 10 degrees to replicate the general surgical inclination of the cup in the pelvis of 45 degrees. Cyclic loading was applied pneumatically. The motion cycles were applied identically across all stations through drive bars in the flexion/extension and internal/external rotation axes. All tests were conducted in 25 per cent newborn calf serum (Harlan Sera-Lab, Loughborough, UK) with 0.1 per cent v/v sodium azide antibacterial agent, and ethylenediamine tetra-acetic acid (EDTA) to inhibit the formation of protein deposits on the bearing surfaces.

The motion and loading cycles applied to the test prostheses did not exactly reproduce the *in vivo* situation, which in any event is subject to many variations, and it was therefore necessary to select 'representative' cycles of these parameters to enable meaningful comparisons to be made between prostheses of differing diameters and clearances. When loading and motion cycles similar to physiological cycles were applied, they were described simply as *'physiological'* simulator cycles. International standards now being prepared recommend that a simplified elliptical vector path in the acetabular cup should be adopted. Such motion has been shown to be significant in determining the wear of polymeric cups and the resulting simulation is known as a *'simplified'* cycle. Full details of each cycle are recorded in reference **(21)**.

4.2.2 The metal-on-metal prostheses

A modern form of total replacement hip joint is shown in Fig. 4.1. The most usual diameter for metal-on-metal joints has been 28 mm and the commercially available Ultima metal-on-metal system (DePuy International, Leeds, UK) was therefore adopted. In order to investigate the effect of femoral head diameter on the lubrication and wear of metal-on-metal prostheses, joints of 16 mm, 22.225 mm (7/8 inch), and 36 mm nominal diameter were also tested in the ten station ProSim simulator described in the previous section. The effects of material differences and variations in surface finish were minimized for joints of all diameters by manufacturing them to the same production standards as the Ultima.

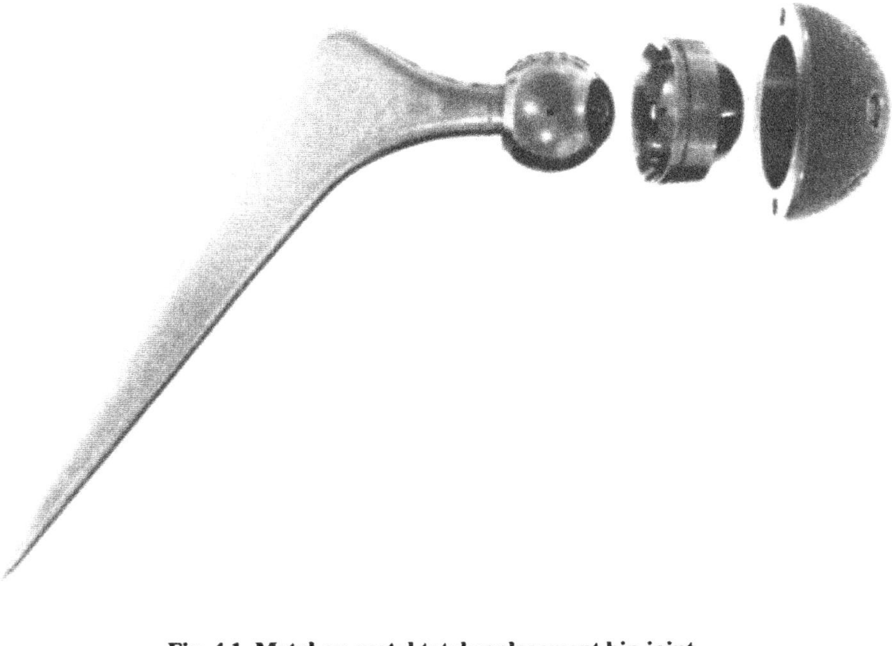

Fig. 4.1 Metal-on-metal total replacement hip joint

Wrought CoCrMo alloy (ASTM F1537) was used with low carbon content (<0.07 per cent) bearing material for the femoral heads and high carbon content (>0.2 per cent) alloy was used for the acetabular cups for the 16 mm, 22.225 mm, and 28 mm joints. The 36 mm joints featured high carbon (>0.2 per cent) heads and cups. An earlier study had shown that there was no significant difference in the wear rate results from the use of either a high- or low-carbon femoral head against a high-carbon acetabular cup **(24)**.

Diametral clearance was measured using a Mitutoyo BHN-506 co-ordinate measuring machine and was about 60 μm for all diameters except the 36 mm prosthesis, where larger diametral clearances ranging from 97 μm to 170 μm were introduced to study the effect of diametral clearance on lubrication and wear.

The surface roughness, R_a, of the femoral heads was measured using a non-contacting interferometer (WYKO RST500, AG Electro Optics, Tarporley, UK), and was on average under 6 nm at manufacture for all head sizes. The acetabular cup surface roughness of the 28 mm and 36 mm joints was also measured using the interferometer. For the smaller joints the interferometer lens was too large to be placed inside the cups, and hence surface roughness was measured using a Taylor Hobson Talysurf. Acetabular roughness, R_a, was initially of the order of 10 nm for all sizes, but the 36 mm cups were rougher, at approximately 30 nm.

4.2.3 Gravimetric technique for wear measurement

Wear of both the femoral and acetabular components was measured gravimetrically using a previously established technique **(25)**. For each measurement the components were extracted from the simulator and bulk contaminants were removed, initially with de-ionized water and then with acetone by wiping the components with a lint-free tissue. The components were then ultrasonically cleaned in a solution of Neutracon detergent, then in de-ionized water. Finally, the components were cleaned with acetone and lint-free tissue. The drying protocol involved placing the cleaned components in an oven at 50 °C and 45 per cent relative humidity for two hours. The components were then placed next to the balance (model MC210S, Sartorius, Epsom, UK) in a controlled environment at 20 °C and 45 per cent relative humidity for two hours prior to weighing. Each component was weighed on the balance, accurate to 0.01 mg, at least three times to find the mean weight. This enabled weight change over the test interval to be determined. Volumetric wear was calculated using a value of 8.33 mg/mm^3 for the density of the CoCrMo alloy. Gravimetric measurements were taken prior to testing, then at various intervals during the test.

4.2.4 Resistivity technique for the detection of lubricating films

The method adopted in this part of the study was to measure the electrical resistance or voltage drop between the femoral head and acetabular cup. This varied considerably, depending upon the presence, or otherwise, of a full or partial separating lubricating film. For metal-on-metal joints this was easy to detect by means of the simple circuit shown in Fig. 4.2. The simple electrical resistivity technique, originally adopted in engineering bearing studies and later applied to metal-on-metal femoral and actebular components has been described elsewhere **(26, 27)**. The metallic femoral and acetabular components were electrically isolated from the simulator using an acetal spacer and nylon screws, and connected by insulated wires which did not interfere with articulation or loading. When the head and cup were completely separated the maximum voltage drop across the joint was 50 mV.

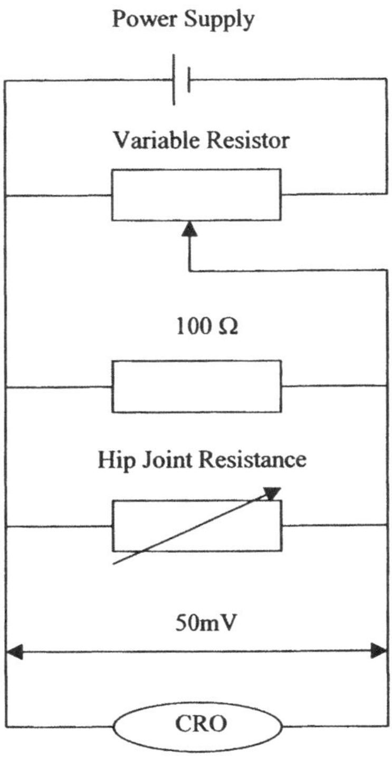

Fig. 4.2 Electrical resistivity circuit used in the lubrication study

When the metallic femoral and acetabular components came into contact a very low electrical resistance resulted. For limited contact between the components, or when extremely thin lubricating films were present, resistance was small and a current passed across the prosthesis. Further separation of the components generated a large electrical resistance and no current flowed. These changes were recorded on a cathode-ray oscilloscope (CRO). To interpret the fluctuations in voltage, and hence lubrication, it was necessary to understand when they occurred during each cycle in relation to motion and load. A dual-channel, storage CRO was therefore used to display load and voltage across the prosthesis simultaneously, and storage of the data was triggered electrically at maximum extension via a non-contacting optical switch. This allowed all variables to be known at any point during each recorded cycle. The stored data was then recorded on a plotter for later analysis.

The lubrication tests ran for approximately 1200 cycles, which was equivalent to about twenty minutes. During testing, CRO traces were typically recorded for the first cycle and after 30, 120, 300, and 1200 cycles.

4.2.5 Iso-viscous elastic lubrication analysis

The possibility of fluid-film lubrication occurring in hard-on-hard total hip replacements during steady walking has been assessed elsewhere **(28, 29)**. The former analysis was based upon the usual assumptions for hydrodynamic lubrication, without any account being taken of elastic deformation of the solids. It was concluded that there was a good possibility of establishing protective fluid films in ceramic-on-ceramic joints and perhaps in some well-finished metal-on-metal implants.

There were two very significant features to the numerical solutions for metal-on-metal joints. In the first place, it was noted that for the joints considered the maximum local elastic deformations (≈ 1–2 μm) were typically about five times greater than the predicted film thicknesses (≈ 0.1–0.3 μm). This indicated that a more complete analysis would have to consider both hydrodynamic and elasticity effects.

The second significant feature of the results of the analysis was that they demonstrated the very powerful effect of squeeze-film action in preserving a near uniform film thickness throughout each cycle, notwithstanding the large variations in load and speed to which the prosthesis was assumed to be subjected. The predicted hydrodynamic film thickness in a 32 mm diameter joint with a small diametral clearance of only 10 μm varied from about 100 to 300 nm.

These findings permit a reasonable estimate to be made of the effective film thickness in metal-on-metal prostheses by assuming that the dominant form of lubrication is the iso-viscous elastic mode of elasto-hydrodynamic lubrication **(30)**. Furthermore, representative mean values of the lubricant viscosity at high shear rates, the applied load, and the entraining velocity can simply be inserted into the appropriate empirical elasto-hydrodynamic film thickness equation.

The minimum film thickness in lubricated, iso-viscous, elastic circular contacts can be estimated from the expression **(30)**

$$H_{min} = \frac{h_{min}}{R} = 2.80 \left(\frac{\eta u}{E'R}\right)^{0.65} \left(\frac{w}{E'R^2}\right)^{-0.21} \tag{4.1}$$

It has been shown in the Notation that the equivalent radius (R) is given, to a very good approximation for all hard-on-hard implants, by the expression ($d^2/2C_d$), and hence it can be seen from equation (4.1) that

$$\begin{aligned}
h_{min} &\propto (\text{lubricant viscosity})^{0.65} \\
&\propto (\text{mean angular velocity})^{0.65} \\
&\propto (\text{head diameter})^{2.19} \\
&\propto (\text{diametral clearance})^{-0.77} \\
&\propto (\text{effective elastic modulus})^{-0.44} \\
&\propto (\text{mean load})^{-0.21}
\end{aligned}$$

For a given lubricant viscosity, kinematic, and loading cycles, the film thickness can be maximized by increasing the femoral head diameter and/or decreasing the diametral clearance and the effective elastic modulus. The latter point explains why, under comparable conditions, the film thickness in metal-on-metal joints exceeds that in ceramic-on-ceramic implants.

4.3 Results

In recent years Goldsmith *et al.* **(25)** and Smith *et al.* **(9, 21)** have recorded the results of wear tests on a number of metal-on-metal implants from a ProSim ten station hip-joint simulator. The detection of lubricating films in similar implants by means of resistivity tests has also been noted by Dowson *et al.* **(27)**, McNie *et al.* **(31)**, and Smith *et al.* **(21)**. These results are now reviewed and analysed under the headings of wear, lubrication, and film thickness.

4.3.1 Wear of metal-on-metal implants

Initially, the wear of four 28 mm and six 36 mm diameter CoCrMo metal-on-metal joints in the simulator was investigated by Goldsmith *et al.* **(25)**. The findings confirmed the remarkably low steady-state wear rate in such joints. While wear rates in the range 30 $mm^3/10^6$ cycles to 100 $mm^3/10^6$ cycles are associated with the more conventional metal-on-polymer joints of diameters 22 mm to 28 mm, the mean wear rates for the 28 mm and 36 mm diameter metal-on-metal joints were only 0.45 $mm^3/10^6$ cycles and 0.36 $mm^3/10^6$ cycles respectively. One of the initial set of three 36 mm diameter joints tested for 5×10^6 cycles exhibited higher wear than the others, resulting in a steady-state wear rate of 0.65 $mm^3/10^6$ cycles, and this was attributed to inadequate fixation in the simulator. Fixation was improved for the final set of three 36 mm joints and these revealed final steady-state wear rates of only 0.07 $mm^3/10^6$ cycles.

Steady-state wear was achieved after about 1×10^6 to 2×10^6 cycles. It was also reported that the heads and cups wore by similar amounts and that the surface roughness of the components tended to converge as running progressed.

Smith *et al.* **(9)** subsequently reported the results of a study of the effect of the femoral head diameter upon wear rate in metal-on-metal joints. Their findings are summarized in Fig. 4.3. As the diameter of the femoral head was increased from 16 mm to 22.225 mm the volumetric wear rate initially increased and was much higher than the wear rates for 28 mm and 36 mm diameter joints. The impressive decline in wear was attributed to the improvement in fluid-film load carrying capacity as the head diameter increased. This indicated that for heads of 28 mm and 36 mm diameter, the mode of lubrication was mixed, with the proportion of load transmitted directly through asperity contacts declining as the diameter increased.

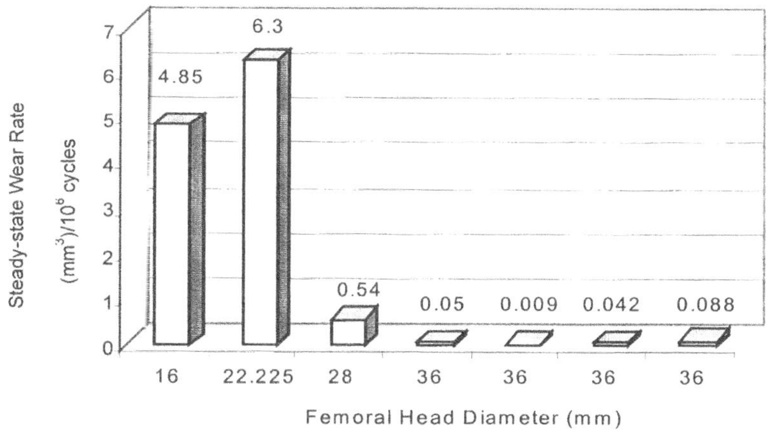

Fig. 4.3 Measured volumetric wear rates for various femoral head diameters when subjected to the simplified walking cycle

The steady-state wear values recorded for the two smallest diameter joints exhibited characteristics of boundary lubrication, since the wear increased as the diameter and hence the sliding distance experienced in each cycle increased. This was consistent with Lancaster's **(32)** wear equation (4.2) in which it can be seen that volumetric wear for fixed wear factors (k) and identical load and angular velocity cycles is directly proportional to sliding distance and hence to head diameter.

$$V = kPx \tag{4.2}$$

The ratio of diameters for the two smaller heads (16/22.225) was 0.72, while that of the wear volumes per unit sliding distance were (4.85/6.30) or 0.77. This measure of agreement between the two ratios is most satisfactory and strongly supportive of a boundary rather than a mixed lubrication regime.

There were thus two modes of lubrication in action; boundary for 16 mm and 22.225 mm joints, and mixed for 28 mm and 36 mm joints. These observations provided a clear indication of the powerful influence of lubrication upon wear in geometrically similar metal-on-metal joints. They also indicated most forcibly that realistic estimates of *in vivo* wear in implants would be achieved from simulator tests only when the tribological conditions were correctly modelled.

Smith *et al.* **(21)** subsequently discussed the wear results in relation to the well known characteristics of journal bearings revealed by the Stribeck friction curve. It was noted that the nature of the observed wear results was consistent with the pattern displayed in Fig. 4.4.

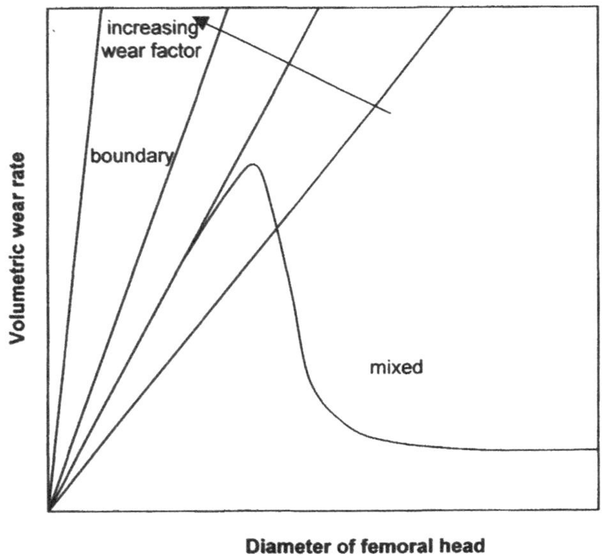

Fig. 4.4 The effect of femoral head diameter upon lubrication and wear in metal-on-metal total hip replacements

4.3.2 Surface contact-separation measurements from the lubrication studies

Voltage-drop measurements based upon the resistivity technique described in Section 4.2.4 were made in separate tests on joints of each of the four diameters used in the wear tests. The 16 mm and 22.225 mm diameter joints showed metallic contact between the femoral and acetabular components at all times during lubrication testing, strongly supporting the indications of boundary lubrication from the wear tests. Due to the steady nature of these traces, the electrical cell was checked pre- and post-test to ensure that the circuit was working correctly. Visual inspection of the bearing surfaces indicated quite clearly that the new components had indeed been in contact, resulting in considerable scratching of the surfaces after only twenty minutes of testing.

The 28 mm diameter joint showed very limited evidence of surface separation during the first few minutes of testing. Some scratching was evident on the bearing surfaces, but this was much smaller than that on the smaller joints.

It was shown in Section 4.2.5 that although head diameter exerted the most powerful effect upon lubricating-film capability, decreasing clearance was also beneficial. The effect of diametral clearance upon lubricating film formation was also investigated for 36 mm diameter joints. The influence of simulated walking cycles, physiological and simplified, was also studied.

The 36 mm diameter joints exhibited differing degrees of surface contact and separation depending upon both diametral clearance and the applied simulated walking cycle. No surface separation was observed for the joint with the largest diametral clearance of 170 μm, for either simulated walking cycle. Surface separation was, however, clearly evident for the smaller clearances from the very first cycle of each test and for both simulated walking cycles. The traces were remarkably consistent in shape over the course of a test and the proportion of surface separation per walking cycle increased as each test progressed. As diametral clearance was reduced the proportion of surface separation in each simulated walking cycle usually increased as shown in Fig. 4.5.

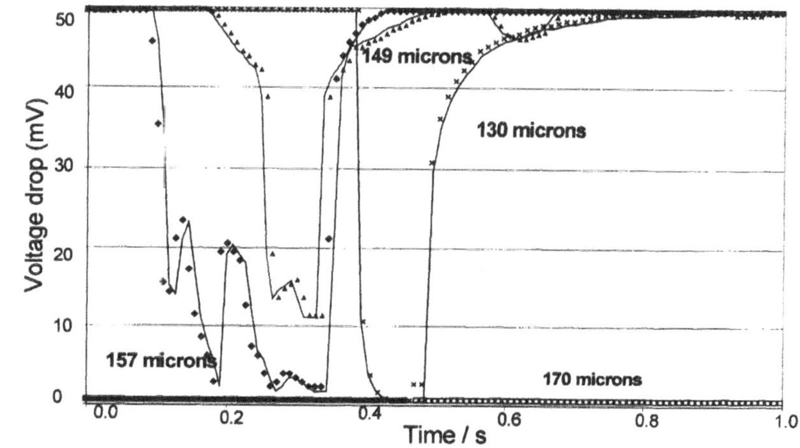

(a) Simplified walking cycle

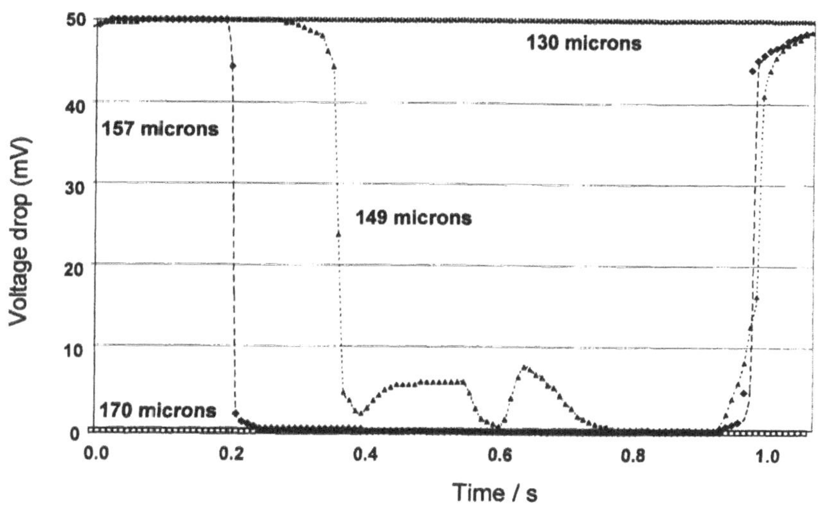

(b) Simulated physiological walking cycle

Fig. 4.5 Resistivity traces for 36 mm diameter joints with a range of diametral clearances

Significantly, a greater proportion of surface separation per walking cycle was observed with the 149 μm and 157 μm diametral clearance joints when subjected to the simplified rather than the physiological cycle. Visual inspection of all the bearing surfaces after testing revealed only a few fine scratches.

The voltage traces exhibited more variability than the wear data, but the trends outlined above were nevertheless quite clear.

4.3.3 Elastohydrodynamic film thickness predictions

In order to shed more light upon the mechanism responsible for the dramatic reduction in wear in metal-on-metal joints illustrated by Fig. 4.3, the elasto-hydrodynamic film thickness for each of the four sizes of implant used in the wear tests has been calculated. It has been shown that the mode of lubrication is iso-viscous-elastic. Following consultation with other research groups, the following *standard* conditions of mean viscosity, load, and angular velocity were adopted.

Lubricant viscosity at high shear rates 0.0009 Ns/m^2
Mean load 2500 N
Mean angular velocity 1.5 rad/s

The corresponding diameters, diametral clearances, calculated film thicknesses, lambda ratios, and measured steady-state wear rates are shown in Table 4.1. The predicted film thickness increases steadily as the implant diameter increases, as shown in Fig. 4.6. There is quite good correlation between film thickness and wear, and it appears that by the time a film thickness of about 12 μm to 14 μm has been established, the wear rate is exceedingly low.

Table 4.1 Influence of joint geometry upon film thickness, lambda ratio, and wear rate (simplified cycle)

Test	*Diameter (mm)*	*Diametral clearance (μm)*	*Theoretical film thickness (nm)*	*Lambda ratio*	*Steady-state wear rate ($mm^3/10^6$ cycles)*
S1	16	61	3.48	0.35	4.85
S2	22.225	56	7.63	0.70	6.30
S3	28	61	11.84	1.97	0.54
S4	36	107	13.32	0.40	0.05
S5	36	125	11.83	0.36	0.009
S6	36	97	14.37	0.80	0.042
S7	36	98	14.25	0.29	0.088

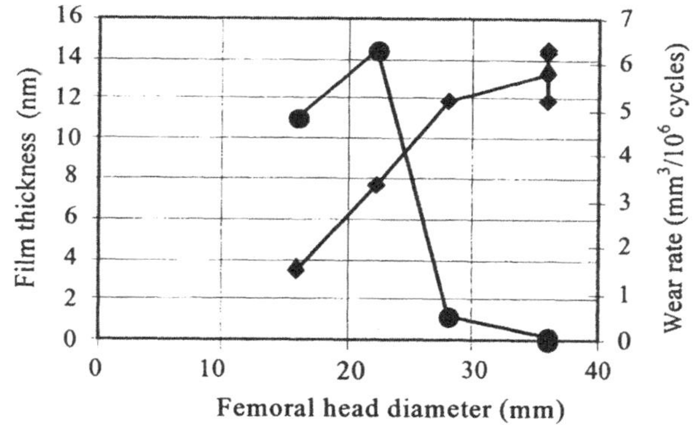

Fig. 4.6 Film thickness and steady-state wear rate (simplified cycle)

In engineering tribology the lambda ratio, representing the ratio of theoretical film thickness to composite surface roughness, has proved to be a useful guide to the performance of highly stressed, lubricated components. If lambda is close to unity there is considerable interaction between asperities. This results in high wear and often premature failure. If values of lambda between two and three can be established, wear is minimized and the life of components can be extended considerably. The lambda ratio does not appear to correlate well with the metal-on-metal hip-joint wear results reported here, although much better correlation was reported by Chan *et al.* **(30)**. In the first place the values of lambda are very low, with six out of seven being less than unity. Figure 4.7 shows little correlation between wear rate and the lambda ratio for the metal-on-metal implants tested. Indeed, the lowest lambda ratios occurred with some of the 36 mm diameter joints which displayed the minimum wear rates. This lack of correlation between lambda and wear rate will be discussed later.

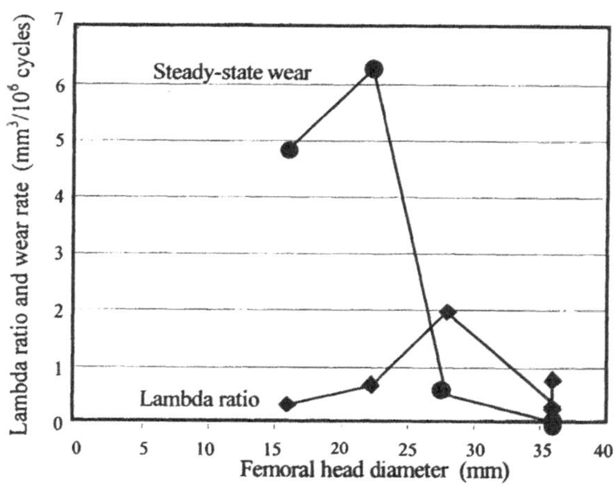

Fig. 4.7 Lambda ratio and steady-state wear rate (simplified cycle)

4.4 Discussion

The simulator wear tests on metal-on-metal total joint replacements reviewed here demonstrate that under certain conditions load-supporting lubricating films can be generated in metal-on-metal joints and that these can exert a powerful effect upon wear. The increasing partial separation of the femoral and acetabular components brought about by increasing diameter and/or reducing clearance, might be attributable to the formation of either boundary or fluid lubricating films. The voltage drop recorded in the experiments initially increased over several seconds, which suggests the development of a boundary lubricating layer, but such films might be expected to promote more uniform separation under all operating conditions. It was also noted that the timing and sequence of the resistivity changes seem to accord better with the concept of fluid-film lubrication. Furthermore, the strong correlation between theoretical elasto-hydrodynamic film thickness and wear rates, reported here and shown in Fig. 4.6, is indicative of fluid-film action. This in turn is determined largely by the femoral head diameter and the diametral clearance.

The two smallest heads clearly operated in the boundary lubrication regime, with the relatively high wear increasing directly with the diameter. This conclusion was also supported by the lack of any detectable voltage drop between the head and the cup.

The benefits resulting from improved lubrication as the head diameter increased were clearly evident, with a substantial reduction in wear taking place between the 22.225 mm and 28 mm diameter head sizes. This reversed the previous trend in which wear increased as the diameter increased. The change also coincided with the initiation of tentative positive voltage drops and hence surface separations during parts of each cycle.

The 36 mm diameter heads developed theoretical elasto-hydrodynamic film thicknesses of the order of 12–14 nm accompanied by even greater reductions in wear. The mean wear rates of about 0.05 $mm^3/10^6$ cycles, measured when the simplified loading cycles were applied to 36 mm diameter joints, were only about 1/140th of the wear rate measured on the 22.225 mm diameter implant.

The voltage traces generally exhibited growing periods of complete or partial separation during each cycle, although there were inevitably some fluctuations in the traces as the rugosities passed through the loaded conjunction. There were very strong indications of increased periods of separation as the diametral clearance was reduced. The most surprising feature of these results was the rapid improvement in the lubrication conditions for relatively small reductions in the diametral clearance. In the 36 mm diameter joint, contact was maintained throughout the cycle at a diametral clearance of 170 μm, while full or partial separation was recorded for most of the cycle when the diametral clearance was reduced by only 40–130μm.

The theoretical elasto-hydrodynamic film thickness was, on average, only 70 per cent of the composite surface roughness, and it exceeded it only once. Furthermore, there was no clear correlation between wear rate and the lambda ratio, as shown by Fig. 4.7. Indeed, the low lambda values representative of the 36 mm diameter joints corresponded to the minimum wear rates recorded. This is, at first sight, surprising since it might reasonably be expected that the ratio of theoretical film thickness to mean asperity height would influence wear directly. However, the original concept of the lambda ratio and the determination of a composite roughness was based upon the assumption of a Gaussian distribution of heights. This is clearly a poor representation of the surfaces of metallic hip-joint components, particularly after wear. There are also indications that material structure, in the form of grain size and carbide distribution, may be important in the wear process. Finally, the simple analysis of wear and lubrication presented here takes no account of the presence of wear debris within the clearance space between the femoral head and the acetabular cup. Third body action must result from the combination of the lubricating film and the wear debris.

The indications from the present study strongly suggest that the predicted elasto-hydrodynamic film thickness alone provides a stronger link with wear in the mixed lubrication regime in metal-on-metal total joint replacements than does the lambda ratio. Indeed, the correlation is sufficiently strong to suggest that a useful design guide could result from the use of equation (4.1) alone. Remarkably low wear rates resulted when the calculated film thickness reached values in the range 12–14 μm in the present tests.

4.5 Conclusions

An analysis of the wear and lubrication studies reported in recent years by Goldsmith, McNie, Smith, and Dowson enables the following conclusions to be drawn.

- The mode of lubrication in metal-on-metal joints is strongly influenced by femoral head diameter and diametral clearance.
- In the joint simulator, joints with relatively small femoral heads of diameter 16 mm and 22.225 mm operated in the boundary lubrication regime, while the performance of joints of 28 mm and 36 mm diameter indicated that mixed lubrication prevailed.
- In the small diameter joints wear rates increased as the head diameter increased. Further increases in the head diameter caused the wear rate to decline continuously as the mixed lubrication regime developed.
- The wear rates in 36 mm diameter metal-on-metal joints tested in the ProSim simulator with a simplified cycle were extremely small, being of the order of 0.05 $mm^3/10^6$ cycles.
- The average wear rate encountered in 36 mm diameter joints was only 1/140th of that recorded for 22.225 mm diameter joints.
- There was good correlation between the predicted elasto-hydrodynamic film thickness and the wear rate in the mixed lubrication regime prevalent in the larger diameter joints.
- For the assumed average conditions of lubricant viscosity, load, and angular velocity, film thicknesses in the range 12–14 μm were predicted in the region of minimum wear. This finding needs to be tested further in relation to results reported by others for different joints and different simulators.
- There was no discernable correlation between wear rate and lambda ratio, thus raising doubts about the value of the latter parameter in metal-on-metal hip-joint design. This finding calls for further investigation. In particular, the influence of non-normal distributions of surface asperities upon the significance of the lambda ratio needs to be investigated.
- The role of material properties, grain size, and carbide distribution upon wear in the mixed lubrication regime in total replacement metal-on-metal joints should be further explored.
- The interaction between lubricant and wear debris in the third-body process between articulating surfaces should be examined.

4.6 Acknowledgement

In the tribological study presented here data revealed in studies carried out and reported by three DePuy International Post-doctoral Research Fellows, Andrew Goldsmith, Catriona McNie, and Simon Smith have been analysed. Appreciation is offered to DePuy International Limited (a Johnson and Johnson Company) for their sponsorship of the Research Fellows and access to the Company research laboratory and the ProSim simulator.

4.7 References

(1) **Dowson, D.** (2001), New joints for the millennium: wear control in total replacement hip joints, Proc. Instn Mech. Engrs, Part H, *Journal of Engineering in Medicine*, **215**, H4, pp 335–358.

(2) **McKee, G. K.** and **Watson-Farrar, J.** (1966) Replacement of arthritic hips by the McKee-Farrar prostheses. *J. Bone Jt. Surg.*, **48-B**, 245–259.

(3) **Amstutz, H.** (1996) Metal-on-metal hip prostheses: past performance and future directions. *Clin. Orthop. Rel. Res.*, **329**, s297–s303.

(4) **Semlitsch, M.** and **Willert, H. G.** (1997) Clinical wear behaviour of ultra-high molecular weight polyethylene cups paired with metal and ceramic ball heads in comparison to metal-on-metal pairings of hip joint replacements. Proc. Instn Mech. Engrs, Part H, *Journal of Engineering in Medicine*, **211**, H1, 73–88.

(5) **Anissian, H. L., Stark, A., Gustafson, Good, V.**, and **Clarke, I. C.** (1999) Metal-on-metal bearing in hip prosthesis generates 100-fold less wear debris than metal-on-polyethylene. *Acta. Orthop. Scand.*, **70**, 6, 578–582.

(6) **Atkinson, J. R., Dowson, D., Isaac, G. H.**, and **Wroblewski, B. M.** (1985) Laboratory wear tests and clinical observations of the penetration of femoral heads into acetabular cups in total replacement hip joints. III: The measurement of internal volume changes in explanted Charnley sockets after 2-16 years *in vivo* and the determination of wear factors. *Wear*, **104**, 225–244.

(7) **Livermore, J., Ilstrup, D.**, and **Morrey, B.** (1990) Effect of femoral head size on wear of the polyethylene acetabular component. *J. Bone Jt Surg.*, **72-A**, 518–528.

(8) **Hall, R. M., Unsworth, A., Siney, P.**, and **Wroblewski, B. M.** (1996) Wear in retrieved Charnley acetabular sockets. Proc. Instn Mech. Engrs, Part H, *Journal of Engineering in Medicine*, **210**, H1, 17–34.

(9) **Smith, S. L., Dowson, D.**, and **Goldsmith, A. A. J.** (2001) The effect of femoral head diameter upon lubrication and wear of metal-on-metal total hip replacements. Proc. Instn Mech. Engrs, Part H, *Journal of Engineering in Medicine*, **215**, H, 161–170.

(10) **Wait, M. E., Walker, P. S.**, and **Blunn, G. W.** (1995) Tissue reaction of CoCr wear debris from metal on metal total hip replacements. *Trans. Eur. Orthop. Res. Soc.*, Munich, Germany, 1995, p 462.

(11) **Soh, E. W., Blunn, G. W., Wait, M. E.**, and **Walker, P. S.** (1996) Size and shape of metal particles from metal on metal total hip replacements. *Trans. 42nd Annual Mtg Orthop. Res. Soc.*, Atlanta, Georgia, p 462.

(12) **Shanbhag, A. S., Jacobs, J. J., Glant, T. T., Gilbert, J. L., Black, J.**, and **Galante, J. O.** (1994) Composition and morphology of wear debris in failed uncemented total hip replacements. *J. Bone Jt Surg.*, **76-B**, 1, 60–67.

(13) **Tipper, J. L., Ingham, E., Hailey, J. L., Besong, A. A., Stone, M., Wroblewski, B. M.**, and **Fisher, J.** (1997) Quantitative comparison of polyethylene wear debris, wear

rate and head damage in retrieved hip prostheses. *Trans. 43rd Annual Mtg Orthop. Res. Soc.*, San Fransico, California, p 355.

(14) **Green, T. R., Fisher, J., Stone, M., Wroblewski, B. M.,** and **Ingham, E.** (1998) Polyethylene particles of a 'critical size' are necessary for the induction of cytokines by macrophages *in vitro*. *Biomaterials*, **19**, 24, 2297–2302.

(15) **Murray, D. W.** and **Rushton, N.** (1990) Macrophages stimulate bone resorption when they phagocytose particles. *J. Bone Jt Surg.*, **72-B**, 988–992.

(16) **Shanbhag, A. S., Jacobs, J. J., Black, J., Galante, J. O.,** and **Glant, T. T.** (1994) Macrophage/particle interactions: effect of size, composition and surface area. *J. Biomed. Mater. Res.*, **28**, 1, 81–90.

(17) **Tabata, Y.** and **Ikada, Y.** (1988) Effect of the size and surface charge of polymer microspheres on their phagocytosis by macrophage. *Biomaterials*, **9**, 4, 356–362.

(18) **Ingham, E.** and **Fisher, J.** (2000) Biological reactions to wear debris in total joint replacement, Proc. Instn Mech. Engrs, Part H, *Journal of Engineering in Medicine*, **214**, H1, 21–37.

(19) **Fisher, J., Bell, J., Barbour, P. S. M., Tipper, J. L., Matthews, J. B., Besong, A. A., Stone, M. H.,** and **Ingham, E.** (2001) A novel method for the prediction of functional biological activity of polyethylene wear debris, Proc. Instn Mech. Engrs, Part H, *Journal of Engineering in Medicine*, **215**, H2, 127–132.

(20) **Endo, M., Tipper, J. L., Barton, D. C., Stone, M. H., Ingham, E.,** and **Fisher, J.** (2002) Comparison of wear, wear debris and functional biological activity of moderately crosslinked and non-crosslinked polyethylenes in hip prostheses Proc. Instn Mech. Engrs, Part H, *Journal of Engineering in Medicine*, **215**, H2, 111–122.

(21) **Smith, S. L., Dowson, D.,** and **Goldsmith, A. A. J.** (2001) The lubrication of metal-on-metal total hip joints: a slide down the Stribeck curve, Proc. Instn Mech. Engrs, Part J, *Journal of Engineering Tribology*, **215**, J5, 483–493.

(22) **Dowson, D.** (1998) *History of Tribology*, (Second Edition), Professional Engineering Publishing Limited, London and Bury St Edmunds, UK, pp 1–768.

(23) **Goldsmith, A. A. J.** and **Dowson, D.** (1999) Development of a ten-station, multi-axis hip joint simulator. Proc. Instn Mech. Engrs, Part H, *Journal of Engineering in Medicine*, **213**, 311–316.

(24) **Firkins, P. J., Tipper, J. L., Ingham, E., Stone, M. H., Farrar, R.,** and **Fisher, J.** (1999) Quantitative analysis of wear debris from metal on metal hip prostheses tested in a physiological hip joint simulator. *Trans. 45th Annual Mtg Orthop. Res. Soc.*, Anaheim, California, p 49.

(25) **Goldsmith, A. A. J., Dowson, D., Isaac, G. H.,** and **Lancaster, J. G.** (2000) A comparative joint simulator study of the wear of metal-on-metal and alternative material combinations in hip replacements. Proc. Instn Mech. Engrs, Part H, *Journal of Engineering in Medicine*, **214**, H1, 39–47.

(26) **Dowson, D., Harrison, P., Taylor, C. M.,** and **Zhu, G.** (1990) Experimental observations of lubricant film state between a cam and bucket follower using the electrical resistivity technique. *Proceedings of the Japan International Tribology Conference*, Nagoya, Japanese Society of Tribologists 1990, 119–124.

(27) **Dowson, D., McNie, C. M.,** and **Goldsmith, A. A. J.** (2000) Direct experimental evidence of lubrication in a metal-on-metal total hip replacement tested in a joint simulator. Proc. Instn Mech. Engrs, Part C, *Journal of Mechancial Engineering Science*, **214**, 75–86.

(28) **Jin, Z. M.** and **Dowson, D.** (1999) A full numerical analysis of hydrodynamic lubrication in artificial hip joints replacements constructed from hard materials. Proc.

Instn Mech. Engrs, Part C, *Journal of Mechancial Engineering Science*, **213**, C4, 355–370.

(29) **Chan, F. W., Medley, J. B., Bobyn, J. D.,** and **Krygier, J. J.** (1998) Time-varying fluid film lubrication of metal-metal hip implants in simulator tests, ORS.

(30) **Hamrock, B. J.** and **Dowson, D.** (1981) Ball bearing lubrication: the elastohydrodynamics of elliptical contacts, John Wiley & Sons, New York, pp 386.

(31) **McNie, C. M.** and **Dowson, D.** (2000) The effect of radial clearance on lubrication in a metal on metal joint tested in a hip joint simulator, in *Proceedings of the 26th Leeds-Lyon Symposium on Tribology*, 'Thinning Films and Tribological Interfaces', Ed. Dowson, D. *et al.*, Elsevier Science B V, 341–345.

(32) **Lancaster, J. K.** (1973) Dry bearings: a survey of materials and factors affecting their performance. *Tribology*, **6**, December 1973, 219–251.

(33) **Chan, F. W., Bobyn, J. D., Medley, J. B., Krygier, J. J.,** and **Tanzer, M. T.** (1999) Wear and lubrication of metal-on-metal hip implants, The Otto Aufranc Award, Clinical Orthopaedics and Related Research, Number 368, 10–24.

D Dowson, A A J Goldsmith, C M McNie, and **S L Smith**
School of Mechanical Engineering, The University of Leeds, UK

5

The Lubrication and Friction of Conventional UHMWPE, Novel Compliant Layer, and Hard Bearing Surfaces for use in Total Hip Prostheses

S C Scholes, S L Smith, H E Ash, and **A Unsworth**

Abstract

Total hip replacement (THR) surgery today generally incorporates a metal or ceramic femoral head articulating against an ultra-high molecular weight polyethylene (UHMWPE) acetabular cup and can be expected to last in excess of fifteen years. The introduction of components which exhibit low wear such as hard bearing surfaces or compliant layer joints could extend the life of THRs. The friction and lubrication properties of conventional metal- and ceramic-on-UHMWPE prostheses, metal-on-metal prostheses, and metal-on-polyurethane compliant layer joints were evaluated both experimentally and theoretically. All of the joint combinations operated in the mixed lubrication regime with compliant layers giving the lowest friction. With further optimization of the design of these compliant layers and hard bearing surface joints, full fluid-film lubrication should be achievable.

Notation

a contact radius
E_{adj} adjusted elastic modulus for layers of $\upsilon_2 > 0.4$
E' equivalent elastic modulus
E'' elastic modulus term
E''' elastic modulus term

E_1	elastic modulus of femoral head
E_2	elastic modulus of acetabular cup
f	friction factor
h_{min}	minimum film thickness
h_t	layer thickness
L	applied load
r	radius of the femoral head
R_c	radius of the acetabular cup
R_x	equivalent radius, $1/R_x = 1/r - 1/R_c$
S_q	average root mean square roughness
S_{q1}	average root mean square roughness of femoral head
S_{q2}	average root mean square roughness of acetabular cup
T	frictional torque
T_i	frictional torque from inverse cycle
T_n	frictional torque from normal cycle
u	entraining velocity = $(u_1 + u_2)/2$
u_1	sliding velocity of the femoral head
u_2	sliding velocity of the acetabular cup
z	Sommerfeld number
η	lubricant viscosity
λ	dimensionless surface separation ratio
υ_1	Poisson's ratio of femoral head
υ_2	Poisson's ratio of acetabular cup

5.1 Introduction

The healthy synovial joint is an exceptional natural bearing which provides low wear and low friction for many decades. Under normal conditions this type of natural joint operates mainly in the full fluid film lubrication regime **(1, 2)**, where the opposing surfaces of the joint are separated by a film of lubricant and any load is carried by the pressure generated within the lubricant (synovial fluid). The fluid film is achieved by a combination of elastohydrodynamic lubrication (EHL), microelastohydrodynamic lubrication (μEHL), and squeeze film lubrication.

Unfortunately diseases, such as osteoarthritis, or injury can destroy this natural bearing system. Total hip replacement (THR) is now regarded as the best and most effective treatment to alleviate the pain, discomfort, and disability caused by diseased or damaged joints. The most popular type of prosthesis used in THR surgery today incorporates a metal or ceramic femoral head which articulates against an ultra-high molecular weight polyethylene (UHMWPE) acetabular cup, such as the Charnley low friction arthroplasty. Currently, an artificial hip prosthesis can be expected to last on average in excess of fifteen years with failure due, in the majority of cases, to late aseptic loosening of the acetabular component **(3, 4)**. Every year, globally, more and more people take advantage of THR surgery and more hip arthroplasties are being performed on the younger patient. The longevity of these joints is therefore becoming increasingly important.

Several theories have been put forward to explain the cause of late aseptic loosening of the acetabular component. The most popular view is that of debris-induced osteolysis (bone resorption) of the periprosthetic bone resulting in failure of the joint at the fixation interface **(5, 6)**. Unlike natural, healthy synovial joints, conventional artificial joints operate in the mixed lubrication regime, where the bearing surfaces are not completely separated and the load is carried partly by the fluid pressure and partly by the contacting asperities **(7–10)**. This contact inevitably results in wear. When wear debris is produced by the implant, whether it be from the articulating surfaces, the bone-cement interface, or any other source, the fibrous tissue layer surrounding the implant will try to expel these 'foreign bodies'. If it is not possible for the body to break down these particles, as is the case for UHMWPE, macrophages or multi-nucleated giant cells (MNGC) will engulf the particles and release cytokines which directly stimulate osteoclastic activity leading to bone resorption and eventually to possible loosening of the implant **(11)**.

It has been found that the size of the wear particle influences the type of tissue reaction. If the particles are large (>5 μm) they are not phagocytosed but are surrounded by MNGC; if the particles are smaller (which is usually the case for polyethylene, metal, and ceramic particles alike) they are engulfed by macrophages **(6, 12, 13)**. Further to this, the macrophage response to wear particles has also been found to be more aggressive to particles in the size range 0.2–8 μm **(14)**.

Another view as to the cause of osteolysis involves loosening due to mechanical factors such as micromotion of the implant, stress shielding, and elevated fluid pressure resulting in resorption rather than the biological response to wear debris. Poor initial stability and fixation of an implant at surgery can lead to micromotion. It has been suggested that it is this micromotion of the implant that causes the osteolysis with the wear particles then inhibiting new bone formation **(15)**.

There is substantial circumstantial evidence in support of the theory of debris-induced bone resorption. Indeed, macrophages containing particulate debris have been found in association with well fixed, stable components **(5)**. Therefore it is likely that both motion of the joint and the biological reaction to the particulate debris are important in the aseptic loosening of artificial hip joints.

A realistic alternative to the problem of wear in conventional metal or ceramic on UHMWPE prostheses is the introduction of bearing surfaces which exhibit low wear that operate in the full fluid-film lubrication regime, which may be achieved either through the development of hard bearing surfaces or compliant layer joints.

A high number of failures led the early metal-on-metal joints (such as the McKee–Farrar prosthesis) to lose favour to the Charnley-type metal-on-UHMWPE prosthesis **(16–18)**. Despite this high incidence of failure, there have been reported cases of success after as many as twenty years of use **(19, 20)**. By designing these new generation metal-on-metal total hip prostheses to tighter tolerances and using superior alloy compositions it is thought that the long term survivorship of metal-on-metal implants can be further and more consistently improved. Jin *et al.* **(21)** concluded that it was possible to achieve full fluid-film lubrication in both metal-on-metal and ceramic-on-ceramic joints provided that the bearing surfaces were smooth enough.

Compliant layer joints are designed to operate in a similar way to the natural synovial joint in that they incorporate a 'compliant' polyurethane layer rather than polyethylene as the acetabular cup bearing surface, thus promoting the joint to enjoy full fluid-film lubrication using both EHL and μEHL.

This study compares the friction and lubrication regimes of conventional metal- and ceramic-on-UHMWPE prostheses with the friction and lubrication regimes of metal-on-metal and the novel metal-on-polyurethane compliant layer joints.

5.2 Materials and methods

Table 5.1 shows the material combinations tested in this study.

Table 5.1 Material combinations tested in this study

Femoral component	*Acetabular component*	*Diameter (mm)*	*Radial clearance (mm)*	*Equivalent radius, R_x (m)*	*Equivalent Elastic modulus, E' (Pa)*
CoCrMo	UHMWPE	28	0.20	0.99	4.7×10^9
Zirconia	UHMWPE	28	0.20	0.99	4.7×10^9
CoCrMo*	Polyurethane*	32	0.25	1.04	n/a
CoCrMo	CoCrMo	28	0.03	6.55	2.1×10^{11}
CoCrMo**	Polyurethane**	32	0.17	1.51	n/a
Al_2O_3**	Al_2O_3**	28	0.03	6.55	3.8×10^{11}

* Two joints of this type were tested with different layer thickness

** These joints were not tested in this study but their parameters are given here for comparison

Frictional measurements of all the joints were carried out on one of the two Durham Hip Function Simulators. In summary, a servohydraulic mechanism controlled by a PC via a microprocessor allowed a dynamic loading cycle similar to that found by English and Kilvington **(22)** to be applied to the joints. The loading cycle had the maximum and minimum loads set at 2000 N and 100 N respectively. A simple harmonic oscillatory motion of ±24 degrees was applied to the femoral head in the flexion/extension plane. The period of motion of each cycle was 1.2 seconds. The simulator comprised a low friction carriage into which the acetabular cup was positioned and an upper moving frame into which the femoral head was fixed; the prosthesis was therefore inverted relative to its position *in vivo*. The acetabular carriage was supported by externally pressurized bearings which provided both a self-centering mechanism and a very low friction axis about which the carriage could rotate due to the frictional torque generated between the bearing surfaces. This rotation was resisted by a Kistler piezoelectric transducer which was calibrated to measure torque. The simulator is described in further detail elsewhere **(23)**.

In order to obtain accurate measurements of friction, both the femoral head and the acetabular cup were adjusted in height to ensure the axis of rotation of the joint was aligned with that of the friction measurement system. Any horizontal misalignment between the rotational axis of the acetabular carriage and acetabular cup which could not be eliminated *in situ* and hence would lead to an additional eccentricity torque was accommodated by performing two runs on each joint, one with the peak loading applied while the head was moving forwards in the cycle (normal run) and another with the peak loading applied while the head was moving backwards in the cycle (inverse run). These loading cycles each produced a frictional torque T_n and T_i respectively from which the true frictional torque was calculated:

$$T = \frac{|T_i| + |T_n|}{2} \tag{5.1}$$

This frictional torque was then converted to friction factor (f) using the equation below **(24)**:

$$f = \frac{T}{rL} \tag{5.2}$$

where T is the frictional torque between the bearing surfaces, r is the femoral head radius and L is the axial load applied across the joint. Friction factor is similar to the coefficient of friction but varies slightly depending on the elastic contact of the hip joint. The frictional torque, load, and angular displacement were measured throughout the loading cycle and an average friction factor was taken from the high load, high velocity stage of the loading cycle (equivalent to the stance phase of walking).

Tests were performed with different viscosities, η, of carboxymethyl cellulose (CMC) fluids ($0.001 < \eta < 0.100$ Pa s). CMC fluids have been shown to have similar rheological properties to synovial fluid, i.e. they are shear-thinning **(25)**. All viscosities were measured on a Ferranti–Shirley cone-on-plate viscometer at a shear rate of 3000 s^{-1} and at room temperature. The joints were tested three times each and were cleaned thoroughly before each test.

Stribeck analysis was used to give an indication of the mode of lubrication, in which friction factor was plotted against Sommerfeld number, z, which was defined as:

$$z = \frac{\eta u r}{L} \tag{5.3}$$

Here, η is the viscosity of the lubricant and u is the entraining velocity of the bearing surfaces. A decrease in friction factor with increase in Sommerfeld number is indicative of a mixed lubrication regime in which the load is carried in part by the contact between the asperities of the bearing surfaces and also by the pressure generated within the lubricant. A rising trend is indicative of a full fluid-film regime where the two surfaces are completely separated by the lubricant film and the frictional resistance is generated solely by the shear within the fluid.

Surface topography measurements were performed using a Zygo NewView 100 non-contacting, three-dimensional profilometer. Five measurements of root mean square roughness, S_q, were taken at random within the presumed contact zone of both the femoral head and the acetabular cup of each material combination.

Due to the importance of the elastic deformation of the surfaces in both the conventional metal- or ceramic-on-polymer joints and the hard bearing surfaces **(21)**, the theory of Hamrock and Dowson **(26)** for low elastic modulus materials was used in predicting the minimum film thickness for these two material combinations.

$$\frac{h_{\min}}{R_x} = 2.798\left(\frac{\eta u}{E'R_x}\right)^{0.65}\left(\frac{L}{E'R_x^2}\right)^{-0.21} \tag{5.4}$$

where h_{min} is the minimum film thickness, R_x is the equivalent radius for a ball on plane model, η is the viscosity of the lubricant [taken as 0.010 Pa s as this is of the same order of magnitude as pathological synovial fluid **(27)**], u is the entraining velocity (maximum of 0.010 ms^{-1} for the Durham Hip Function Simulator), E' is the equivalent elastic modulus of the material pairing, and L is the applied axial load across the joint (2000 N).

$$\frac{1}{E'} = 0.5\left\{\left(\frac{1-\upsilon_1^2}{E_1}\right)+\left(\frac{1-\upsilon_2^2}{E_2}\right)\right\} \tag{5.5}$$

where υ_1 and E_1 are the Poisson's ratio and elastic modulus of the head respectively, and υ_2 and E_2 are the Poisson's ratio and elastic modulus of the cup respectively.

The film thicknesses for the compliant layer joints were calculated from the theory of Dowson and Yao **(28)**.

$$h_{\min} = 1.59R_x\left(\frac{\eta u}{E''R_x}\right)^{0.56}\left(\frac{h_t E''}{E'''R_x}\right)^{0.36}\left(\frac{L}{E''R_x^2}\right)^{-0.20} \tag{5.6}$$

where η, u, and L have the same values as for the conventional joints and hard bearing surfaces above, h_t is the compliant layer thickness (3.5 mm and 3 mm for joints 1 and 2 respectively), and R_x for these compliant layer joints is shown in Table 5.1. The constrained column model, used to derive the above formula, is restricted to compliant materials with a Poisson's ratio of less than 0.4, whereas the polyurethanes used as the layer in compliant layer joints have a Poisson's ratio approaching 0.5. In order to accommodate a layer of $\upsilon_2 = 0.5$, Dowson *et al.* **(29)** indicated that an adjusted modulus, E_{adj}, should be used thus allowing the film thickness equations based on the constrained column model to be applied to incompressible layers.

$$E_{adj} = \frac{4LR_x h_t}{\pi a^4}\left\{\frac{(1+\upsilon_2)(1-2\upsilon_2)}{1-\upsilon_2}\right\} \tag{5.7}$$

where a is the contact radius given by:

$$a = 0.94h_t^{0.38}\left(\frac{LR_x}{E_2}\right)^{0.21} \tag{5.8}$$

where E_2 is the elastic modulus of the compliant layer (30 MPa). The modulus terms E'' and E''' are given by:

$$\frac{1}{E''} = \frac{1-\upsilon_2^2}{E_{adj}} \qquad (5.9)$$

and

$$\frac{1}{E'''} = \frac{(1+\upsilon_2)(1-2\upsilon_2)}{(1-\upsilon_2)E_{adj}} \qquad (5.10)$$

where $\upsilon_2 = 0.4$ throughout.

The predicted minimum film thicknesses, together with the recorded values of S_{q1} and S_{q2}, the average root mean square roughnesses of the head and the cup respectively, were used to determine the dimensionless parameter λ **(30)** and therefore the theoretical lubrication regimes acting within the joints for all of the material combinations.

$$\lambda = \frac{h_{\min}}{\left(S_{q1}^2 + S_{q2}^2\right)^{0.5}} \qquad (5.11)$$

Experimental observation shows that if the ratio of the minimum film thickness to the combined surface roughness, λ, is less than three then mixed lubrication is likely. If $\lambda > 3$ then a full fluid-film lubrication regime is predicted **(30)** where the asperities of the bearing surfaces are completely separated by the lubricant film.

5.3 Results

The surface roughness values of each femoral head and acetabular cup are shown in Table 5.2.

Table 5.2 Surface roughness values for the joints tested in this study

Joint type	*Femoral S_{q1} (nm)*	*Acetabular S_{q2} (nm)*
CoCrMo/UHMWPE	4.2	279
Zirconia/UHMWPE	3.7	279
CoCrMo/Polyurethane (joint 1)	8.0	163
CoCrMo/Polyurethane (joint 2)	5.0	163
CoCrMo/CoCrMo	8.0	80

5.3.1 Conventional metal- and ceramic-on-UHMWPE joints

The Stribeck curves for the CoCrMo-on-UHMWPE and zirconia-on-UHMWPE joints are shown in Fig. 5.1. Both joints show a general decrease in friction factor with increasing Sommerfeld number, indicative of the mixed lubrication regime with friction factors ranging from 0.04 at the lower viscosities to 0.01 at the higher viscosities. All the points on this curve are to the left of the λ

= 3 line, also suggesting a mixed lubrication regime. Theoretically, for these joints, the transition from mixed lubrication to full fluid film lubrication should occur at a viscosity of 0.38 Pa s. A typical value for the viscosity of pathological synovial fluid is 0.01 Pa s at 3000 s^{-1}.

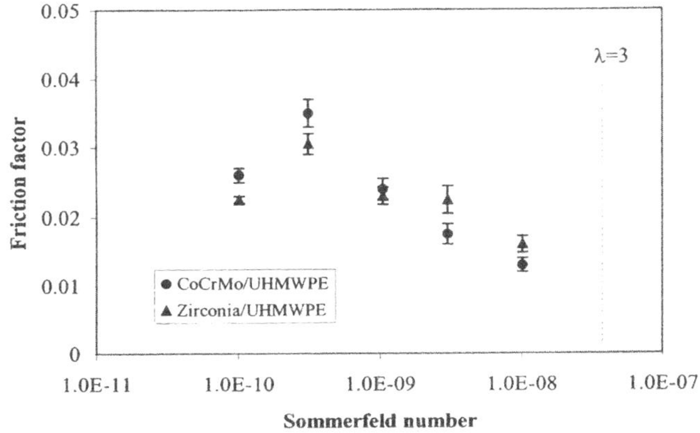

Fig. 5.1 Stribeck plot for the conventional metal- and ceramic-on-UHMWPE joints

5.3.2 Metal-on-polyurethane compliant layer joints

Figure 5.2 shows the Stribeck curves for both of the soft layer joints tested. The friction factors produced by both joints were extremely low (range 0.012–0.001). The friction factors of 0.001 at the higher end of the viscosity range were indicative of full fluid-film lubrication. Indeed, theory would suggest that the transition from mixed to full fluid-film lubrication should occur at a viscosity of 0.03 Pa s, a value much lower than that for the conventional UHMWPE joints.

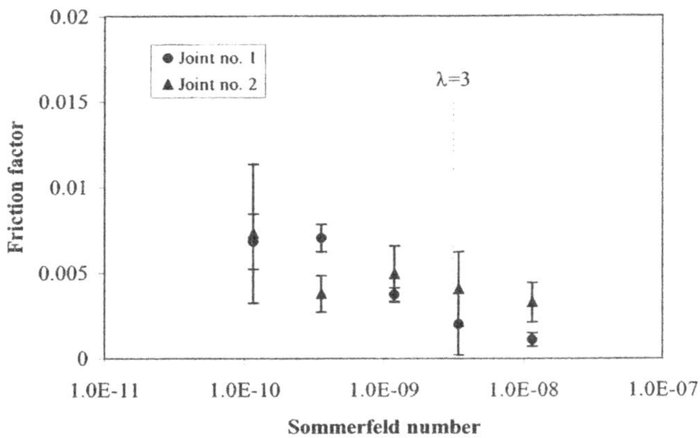

Fig. 5.2 Stribeck plot for polyurethane compliant layer joints numbers 1 and 2

5.3.3 Hard metal bearing surface joints

The Stribeck plot for the CoCrMo-on-CoCrMo joint can be seen in Fig. 5.3. The friction factors produced by this all-metal bearing are high (0.3–0.18). The general trend of a falling friction factor with increasing Sommerfeld number along with the high values of friction is indicative of the mixed lubrication regime. The theory for this type of joint would suggest a transition from mixed to full fluid-film lubrication at a viscosity of 0.079 Pa s.

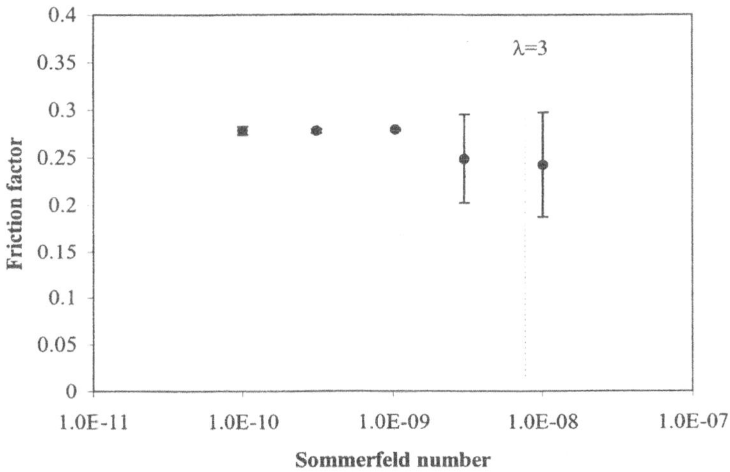

Fig. 5.3 Stribeck plot for the metal-on-metal joint

5.4 Discussion

5.4.1 Conventional metal- and ceramic-on-UHMWPE joints

The friction factors for the conventional metal- and ceramic-on-UHMWPE joints were similar to those found previously by other workers **(7–9, 31–34)**. There was little difference between the results for the two different femoral head materials with the friction factors for the ceramic head being only slightly lower than those with the metal head. This is to be expected as the majority of the friction produced at the bearing surfaces will be due to shearing of the UHMWPE component asperities. The slight reduction in friction factor with the ceramic counterface may be due to the better wettability and surface finish of the ceramic surface **(35)**. This is in agreement with earlier work by Unsworth *et al.* **(36)** and Saikko **(37)**.

Because these joints operate in the mixed lubrication regime wear will occur at the contacting asperities. From Fig. 5.1 it can be seen that in order for these joints to undergo the transition from mixed to full fluid-film lubrication the Sommerfeld number at which the joints operate must be increased. It is not possible to increase the viscosity of the lubricating fluid present within the body, nor is it possible to alter significantly the load to which the joint is subjected. Aside from Sommerfeld number, it is also unlikely that the surface roughnesses of currently manufactured super finished heads will be much further reduced. The only way, therefore, to attain full fluid-film lubrication without changing the bearing materials would be to increase the bearing diameter. However, under the current operating conditions the diameter would need to be increased to 74 mm to achieve this and such a joint diameter is too large to be accommodated by the average human pelvis. It would seem, therefore, that these joints are destined to work in the mixed lubrication regime and that wear is an inevitability. This wear must be reduced to prolong the implant life of these joints. This can be achieved to different extents by either reducing the bearing radius (as since wear in the mixed lubrication regime is related to head size, a smaller diameter head would result in a decreased sliding distance per articulation and therefore a decrease in wear volume), or by using a different type of polyethylene such as cross-linked polyethylene. However, if the joint radius is decreased too much then factors other than wear become important to the longevity of the prosthesis, such as impingement, dislocation, and neck strength.

5.4.2 Metal-on-polyurethane compliant layer joints

For compliant layer joints to work well they must operate within the full fluid-film lubrication regime through the effects of EHL and µEHL in order to reduce both the wear and friction by eliminating the asperity contact between the bearing surfaces. In this study, full fluid-film lubrication was achieved at the higher viscosities; this has also been found by other workers **(38–40)**. Also, due to the high dry friction (circa 1) exhibited by these compliant layer joints it has been shown that minimal asperity contact occurs (less than 1 per cent asperity contact is required to produce the friction factors seen here), even at the low lubricant viscosities **(41)**. Indeed, using a different design of compliant layer joint, Burgess **(41)** found very low friction and full fluid-film lubrication (Fig. 5.4) below the value of Sommerfeld number that theory would suggest for $\lambda = 3$. The hardness of the polyurethane layer has been shown to influence the friction produced by this type of joint greatly **(7)**. This material property is very difficult to reproduce but it is clear that this must be an important factor in the design of such joints.

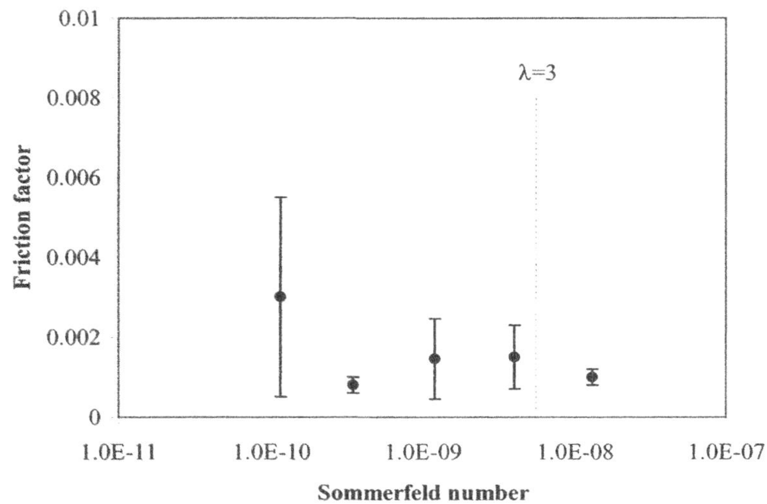

Fig. 5.4 Stribeck plot for polyurethane compliant layer joint (41)

An increase in the bearing radius of this type of joint would result in higher entraining velocities and therefore the transition from mixed to full fluid-film lubrication would occur at viscosities similar to those found in the body. This may lead to very low clinical wear rates.

5.4.3 Hard bearing surfaces

Metal-on-metal joints have, in the past, been shown to operate in the mixed lubrication regime with higher friction than conventional joints **(7, 9, 24, 42)**; this was also found in the present study. Theory suggested a transition from mixed to full fluid-film lubrication within the viscosities tested in this study but this was not confirmed experimentally. The friction factors of 0.25 produced at the viscosity required theoretically to produce full fluid-film lubrication were still high, indicating some asperity contact. This could be due to scratching of the surfaces occurring as a result of mixed lubrication at the lower viscosity lubricants. The increase in surface roughness would result in a shift in the position of the $\lambda = 3$ line to the right of its original position and hence fluid-film lubrication would be expected to occur at a higher viscosity. Friction factors of 0.25 are, however, unlikely to cause loosening of the joint **(43)**.

Hard bearing couplings rely on very smooth surfaces to increase the film thickness to combined surface roughness ratio in order to achieve full fluid-film lubrication. From Figs 5.5 and 5.6 it is clear that a reduction in radial clearance and improved surface roughness will encourage full fluid-film lubrication. The data point representative of the metal-on-metal joints tested in this study is shown on both figures. If the equivalent surface roughness was improved to 0.02 μm then full fluid-film lubrication should be achievable under these operating conditions. The ceramic-on-ceramic joints reported in the study by Scholes and Unsworth **(9)** emphasize this point (Fig. 5.7). These joints were of a high quality surface finish and, when tested under the same conditions as those used in this study, they operated within the full fluid-film lubrication regime with extremely low friction factors. Ceramic-on-ceramic joints also benefit from higher scratch resistance properties and better wettability and therefore enhanced lubrication properties over the metal-on-metal joints. Another advantage of hard bearing combinations for use in hip joint prostheses is their exceptional wear performance. Both metal-on-metal and ceramic-on-ceramic joints have been shown by various workers to exhibit very low wear indeed, with typically one hundredth of the wear of conventional metal- or ceramic-on-UHMWPE joints **(16, 17, 20, 44–50)**.

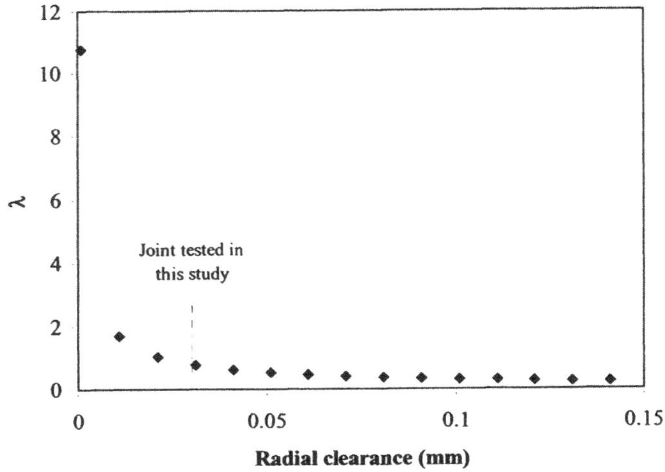

Fig. 5.5 The effect of radial clearance on λ for the metal-on-metal joints (material properties as in Tables 5.1 and 5.2)

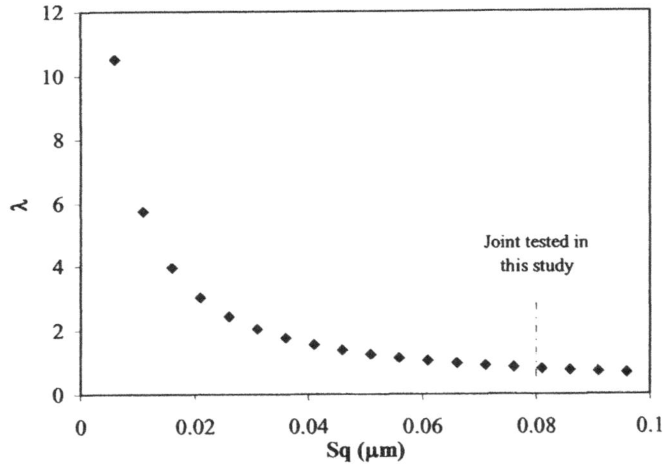

Fig. 5.6 The effect of surface roughness on λ for the metal-on-metal joints (material properties as in Tables 5.1 and 5.2)

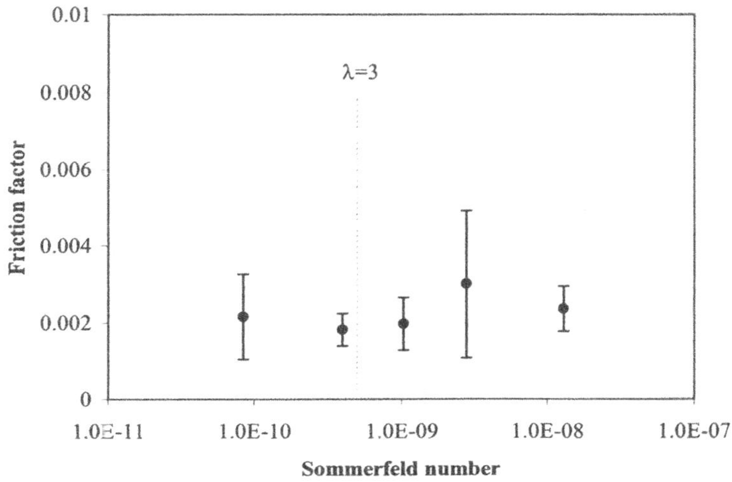

Fig. 5.7 Stribeck plot for ceramic-on-ceramic joints (9)

5.5 Conclusions

Both the compliant layer joints tested in this study and the ceramic-on-ceramic joints tested in a previous study **(9)** gave significantly lower friction than the conventional metal- or ceramic-on-UHMWPE joints. The metal-on-metal joints gave the highest friction of all the joint combinations tested. At the lower lubricant viscosities (those close to the viscosity of synovial fluid) all the joint combinations operated in the mixed lubrication regime and therefore wear (of differing degrees) will occur. The design of the compliant layer joints and the hard bearing surface joints must therefore be optimized to encourage these joints to work in the full fluid-film lubrication regime and hence avoid the problem of wear.

Acknowledgements

The authors would like to thank Stryker Howmedica Osteonics, Biomet Merck Limited, and EPSRC for funding this research.

References

(1) **Unsworth, A., Dowson, D.,** and **Wright, V.** Some new evidence on human joint lubrication. *Ann. Rheum. Dis.*, 1975, **34,** No. 4, 277–285.

(2) **Unsworth, A** and **Amis, A. A.** Biomechanics of articulations and derangements in Disease. In: *Oxford Textbook of Rheumatology*, 1998, Maddison *et al.* eds., second edition, Oxford University Press, 477–485.

(3) **Wroblewski, B. M.** and **Siney, P. D.** Charnley low-friction arthroplasty of the hip – long term results. *Clin. Orthop. Rel. Res.*, 1993, **292**, 191–201.

(4) **Callaghan, J. J., Forest, E. E., Olejniczak, J. P., Goetz, D. D.,** and **Johnston, R. C.** Charnley total hip arthroplasty in patients less than fifty years old. *J. Bone Jt Surg.* 1998, **80-A**, 5, 704–714.

(5) **Howie, D. W., Vernon-Roberts, B., Oakeshott, R.,** and **Manthey, B.** A rat model of resorption of bone at the cement-bone interface in the presence of polyethylene wear particles. *J. Bone Jt Surg.*, 1988, **70-A**, 2, 257–263.

(6) **Schmalzried, T. P., Jasty, M.,** and **Harris, W. H.** Periprosthetic bone loss in total hip arthroplasty. *J. Bone Jt Surg.*, 1992, **74-A**, 6, 849–863.

(7) **Unsworth, A., Pearcy, M. J., White, E. F. T.,** and **White, G.** Frictional properties of artificial hip joints. *J. Engng. in Medicine.*, 1988, **17**, 3, 101–104.

(8) **Unsworth, A.** Tribology of human and artificial joints. *J. Engng. in Medicine.*, 1991, **205**, 163–172.

(9) **Scholes, S. C.** and **Unsworth, A.** Comparison of friction and lubrication of different hip prostheses. *Proc. Instn. Mech. Engrs*, 2000, **214H**, 49–57.

(10) **Wang, A., Essner, A.,** and **Klein, R.** Effect of contact stress on friction and wear of ultra-high molecular weight polyethylene in total hip replacement. *Proc. Instn. Mech. Engrs*, 2001, **215**, H2, 133–139.

(11) **Revell, P. A., AL-Saffar, N.,** and **Kobayashi, A.** Biological reaction to debris in relation to joint prostheses. *Proc. Instn. Mech. Engrs*, 1997, **211**, H2, 187–199.

(12) **Howie, D. W., Manthey, B., Hay, S.,** and **Vernon-Roberts, B.** The synovial response to intraarticular injection in rats of polyethylene wear particles. *Clin. Orthop. Rel. Res.*, 1993, 352–357.

(13) **Schmalzried, T. P., Jasty, M., Rosenberg, A.,** and **Harris, W. H.** Polyethylene wear debris and tissue reactions in knee as compared to hip replacement prostheses. *Journal of Applied Biomaterials*, 1994, **5**, 185–190.

(14) **Green, T. R., Matthews, J. B., Wroblewski, B. M., Fisher, J.,** and **Ingham, E.** Polyethylene particles of a 'critical size' are necessary for the induction of cytokines by macrophages *in vitro*. Presented at the Spring Meeting of the British Orthopaedic Research Society, March 1997.

(15) **Aspenberg, P.** and **Herbertsson, P.** Periprosthetic bone resorption: particles versus movement. *J. Bone Jt Surg.* 1996, **78-B**, 4, 641–646.

(16) **Schmidt, M., Weber, H.,** and **Schön, R.** Cobalt chromium molybdenum metal combination for modular hip prostheses. *Clin. Orthop. Rel. Res.*, 1996, **329S**, S35–S47.

(17) **Kothari, M., Bartel, D. L.,** and **Booker, J. F.** Surface geometry of retrieved McKee-Farrar total hip replacements. *Clin. Orthop. Rel. Res.*, 1996, **329S**, S141–S147.

(18) **Müller, M. E.** The benefits of metal-on-metal total hip replacements. *Clin. Orthop. Rel. Res.*, 1995, **311**, 54–59.

(19) **Jacobsson, S-A., Djerf, K.,** and **Wahlström, O.** 20-year results of McKee-Farrar versus Charnley prosthesis. *Clin. Orthop. Rel. Res.*, 1996, **329S**, S60–S68.

(20) **Schmalzried, T. P., Peters, P. C., Maurer, B. T., Bragdon, C. R.,** and **Harris, W. H.** Long-duration metal-on-metal total hip arthroplasties with low wear of the articulating surfaces. *J Arthroplasty*, 1996, **11**, 3, 322–331.

(21) **Jin, Z. M., Dowson, D.,** and **Fisher, J.** Analysis of fluid film lubrication in artificial hip joint replacements with surfaces of high elastic modulus. *Proc. Instn. Mech. Engrs*, 1997, **211**, 247–256.

(22) **English, T. A.** and **Kilvington, M.** In vivo records of hip loads using a femoral implant with telemetric output (a preliminary report). *J. Biomed. Eng.* 1979, **1**, 2, 111–115.

(23) **Hall, R. M., Unsworth, A., Wroblewski, B. M.,** and **Burgess, I. C.** Frictional characterisation of explanted Charnley hip prostheses. *Wear*, 1994, **175**, 159–166.

(24) **Unsworth, A.** The effects of lubrication in hip joint prostheses. *Phys. Med. Biol.*, 1978, **23**, 2, 253–268.

(25) **Cooke, A. F., Dowson, D.,** and **Wright, V.** The rheology of synovial fluid and some potential synthetic lubricants for degenerate synovial joints. *J. Engng. in Medicine.*, 1978, **7**, 66–72.

(26) **Hamrock, B. J.** and **Dowson, D.** Elastohydrodynamic lubrication of elliptical contacts for materials of low elastic modulus I-Fully flooded conjunction. *J. Lubrication. Technol.*, 1978, **100**, 236–245.

(27) **Scholes, S. C., Unsworth, A.,** and **Goldsmith, A. A. J.** A frictional study of total hip joint replacements. *Phys. Med. Biol.*, 2000, **45**, 12, 3721–3735.

(28) **Dowson, D.** and **Yao, J. Q.** Elastohydrodynamic lubrication of soft-layered solids at elliptical contacts. Part 2: film thickness analysis. *Proc. Instn. Mech. Engrs*, 1994, **208J**, 43–52.

(29) **Dowson, D., Fisher, J., Jin, Z-M., Auger, D. D.,** and **Jobbins, B.** Design considerations for cushion form bearings. *Proc. Instn. Mech. Engrs*, 1991, **205**, 59–68.

(30) **Johnson, K. L., Greenwood, J. A.,** and **Poon, S. Y.** A simple theory of asperity contact in elastohydrodynamic lubrication. *Wear*, 1972, **19**, 91–108.

(31) **Walker, P. S.** Friction of internal artificial joints. *J. Engng. in Medicine.*, 1971, **1**, 4, 91–95.

(32) **Unsworth, A., Dowson, D., Wright, V.,** and **Koshal, D.** The frictional behaviour of human synovial joints – part II: Artificial joints. *Trans. A.S.M.E. J. Lubrication. Technol.*, 1975, July, 377–382.

(33) **O'Kelly, J., Unsworth, A., Dowson, D.,** and **Wright, V.** An experimental study of the friction and lubrication in hip prostheses. *J. Engng. in Medicine.*, 1979, **8**, 3, 153–159.

(34) **Gore, T. A., Higginson, G. R.,** and **Kornberg, R. E.** Some evidence of squeeze-film lubrication in hip prostheses. *J. Engng. in Medicine.*, 1981, **10**, 2, 89–95.

(35) **Smith, S. L., Elfick, A. P. D.,** and **Unsworth, A.** An evaluation of the tribological performance of zirconia and CoCrMo femoral heads. *J Mats. Science*, 1999, **34**, 5159–5162.

(36) **Unsworth, A., Hall, R. M., Burgess, I. C., Wroblewski, B. M., Streicher, R. M.,** and **Semlitsch, M.** Frictional resistance of new and explanted artificial hip joints. *Wear*, 1995, **190**, 226–231.

(37) **Saikko, V.** A simulator study of friction in total replacement joints. *Proc. Instn. Mech. Engrs*, 1992, **206**, 201–211.

(38) **Unsworth, A., Pearcy, M. J., White, E. F. T.,** and **White, G.** Soft layer lubrication of artificial hip joints. *Proc. Instn. Mech. Engrs*, 1987, 715–724.

(39) **Auger, D. D., Dowson, D., Fisher, J.,** and **Jin, Z-M.** Friction and lubrication in cushion form bearings for artificial hip joints. *Proc. Instn. Mech. Engrs*, 1993, **207**, 25–33.

(40) **Smith, S. L., Ash, H. E.,** and **Unsworth, A.** A tribological study of UHMWPE acetabular cups and polyurethane compliant layer cups. *J. Biomed. Mater. Res.: Applied Biomaterials*, 2000, **53**, 710–716.

(41) **Burgess, I. C.** Tribological and mechanical properties of compliant bearings total joint replacements. PhD Thesis, 1996, University of Durham.

(42) **Dowson, D., McNie, C. M.,** and **Goldsmith, A. A. J.** Direct experimental evidence of lubrication in a metal-on-metal total hip replacement tested in a joint simulator. *Proc. Instn. Mech. Engrs Part C*, 2000, **214**, 75–86.

(43) **Andersson, G. B. J., Freeman, M. A. R.,** and **Swanson, S. A. V.** Loosening of the cemented acetabular cup in total hip replacement. *J. Bone Jt Surg.*, 1972, **54B**, 590–599.

(44) **Walter, I. A.** On the material and the tribology of alumina-alumina couplings for hip joint prostheses. *Clin. Orthop. Rel. Res.*, 1992, **282**, 31–46.

(45) **Semlitsch, M.** CoCrMoC metal/metal articulation as a solution to the problem of wear of hip joint replacements. SERC/IMechE Annual Expert Meeting on *Failure of Joint Prostheses,* 28–30 November 1993, 40–45.

(46) **McKellop, H., Park, S. H., Chiesa, R., Doorn, P., Lu, B., Normand, P., Grigoris, P.,** and **Amstutz, H.** In vivo wear of 3 types of metal on metal hip prostheses during 2 decades of use. *Clin. Orthop. Rel. Res.*, 1996, **329S**, S128–S140.

(47) **Chan, F. W., Bobyn, J. D., Medley, J. B., Krygier, J. J., Yue, S.,** and **Tanzer, M.** Engineering issues and wear performance of metal on metal hip implants. *Clin. Orthop. Rel. Res.*, 1996, **333**, 96–107.

(48) **Saikko, V.** and **Pfaff, H-G.** Low wear and friction in alumina/alumina total hip joints. *Acta. Orthop. Scand.*, 1998, **69** (5), 443–448.

(49) **Scholes, S. C., Green, S, M.,** and **Unsworth, A.** The wear of metal-on-metal total hip prostheses measured in a hip simulator. *Proc. Instn. Mech. Engrs*, 2001, **215H**, 523–530.

(50) **Smith, S. L.** and **Unsworth, A.** An in vitro wear study of alumina-alumina total hip prostheses. *Proc. Instn. Mech. Engrs*, 2001, **215H**, 443–446.

S C Scholes, H E Ash, and **A Unsworth**
Centre for Biomedical Engineering, University of Durham, UK
S L Smith
Centre for Design Research, University of Northumbria, Newcastle-upon-Tyne, UK (previously at the Centre for Biomedical Engineering, University of Durham, UK)

6

Prediction of Lubricating Film Thickness in UHMWPE Hip Joint Replacements

Z M Jin, M Jagatia, and D Jalali-Vahid

Abstract

The minimum film thickness has been predicted, based on the elastohydrodynamic lubrication mechanism for a ball-in-socket model with a layered surface, for artificial hip joints employing UHMWPE cups. Various comparisons of the predicted minimum film thickness have been made between ball-in-socket and ball-on-plane models; different bearing surfaces and elasticity models; loading direction and steady-state and transient conditions. A relatively small difference in the minimum film thickness has been predicted between different models under steady-state conditions. The minimum film thickness under cyclic conditions can be accurately estimated by the steady-state model using average values of the load and speed.

Notation

c	Radial clearance, R_2-R_1
C	Displacement coefficients calculated from the finite element method
d	Thickness of UHMWPE acetabular cup, R_3-R_2
E	Modulus of elasticity for UHMWPE bearing surface
f_x, f_y, f_z	Calculated load components defined in equation (6.4)
h	Film thickness
p	Pressure
R_1	Femoral head radius
R_2	Socket radius
R_3	Outside radius of the socket

t	Time
u	Sliding velocity for the ball-on-plane model, ωR_1
w_x, w_y	Components of applied load (w) in the x, y directions respectively
α	Load angle shown in Fig. 6.1(b)
δ	Elastic deformation
ϕ, θ	Angular coordinates in the entraining and side-leakage directions respectively as shown in Fig. 6.1(a)
η	Viscosity of synovial fluid
ν	Poisson's ratio
ω	Angular velocity about the z axis as shown in Fig. 6.1(a).

6.1 Introduction

The major limiting factor to the long-term successful functioning of artificial hip joint replacements is loosening of the implant. The main cause for the loosening has been shown to be osteolysis, resulting from the adverse tissue reaction to wear particles [see **(1)** for a recent review]. Therefore, eliminating or minimizing wear particles offers the key to the long-term success of artificial hip joint replacements. The wear particles are mainly generated at the articulating surfaces through asperity contacts associated with either boundary or mixed lubrication regimes **(2, 3)**. Therefore one of the most effective methods to eliminate or minimize wear particle generation is to reduce asperity contacts between the two bearing surfaces by improving fluid-film lubrication. Under ideal lubrication conditions where the two articulating surfaces are completely separated by a continuous lubricant film, minimum wear can be expected. However, this ideal situation may be very difficult to achieve in artificial hip joint replacements, due to the large dynamic loading and slow speed during walking, as well as start-up and stopping often experienced in the hip joint. Under this later condition, a mixture of both fluid-film lubrication and boundary lubrication or a mixed lubrication regime dominates. Improving the fluid-film formation can reduce the severity of the asperity contact and should theoretically lead to a reduction in wear. It is therefore important to consider lubrication analysis in the design of artificial hip joint replacements. The purpose of this study was to analyse the formation of an elastohydrodynamic lubricating film in artificial hip joint replacements employing a metallic or ceramic femoral ball articulating against an ultra high molecular weight polyethylene (UHMWPE) acetabular socket, and in particular to examine the effect of the following parameters on the predicted lubricating film thickness.

- UHMWPE layer.
- Ball-in-socket geometry.
- Elasticity models for the UHMWPE acetabular cup.
- Direction of loading.
- Transient conditions experienced during walking.

6.2 Lubrication model

An artificial hip joint replacement is often described as a ball-in-socket configuration, consisting of a femoral ball in articulation with an acetabular cup as shown in Fig. 6.1(a). The important geometric parameters are the radii of both the femoral head and the acetabular cup

(R_1 and R_2). There are many forms of bearing couples used for artificial hip joint replacements. The most common one is the combination of a metallic or ceramic femoral head and an UHMWPE acetabular cup. The UHMWPE cup is either fixed to a metallic backing or cemented to the acetabular bone.

The load and speed experienced in the hip joint during steady state walking are dynamic, with an average load of up to 3 to 4 times bodyweight and an average angular velocity as low as 1 rad s^{-1} **(4)**. The lubricant in healthy natural synovial joints is synovial fluid and in total joint replacements is similar to synovial fluid obtained from patients with osteo-arthritis **(5, 6)**. Laboratory measurements of the viscosity–shear rate relationship for synovial fluid have revealed non-Newtonian shear thinning characteristics, particularly at shear rates below 10^3 s^{-1} **(7)**. However, the non-Newtonian synovial fluid behaves reasonably like a Newtonian fluid at the very high shear rates which are likely to be experienced in artificial hip replacements under steady walking conditions **(3)**. Furthermore, the major piezo–viscous effect observed for mineral oils does not appear to be significant for synovial fluid for pressures up to 100 MPa **(7)**, which is unlikely to be exceeded in the UHMWPE hip joint replacement **(8)**. Therefore, the synovial fluid in the present analysis was assumed to be a Newtonian, iso-viscous, and incompressible fluid.

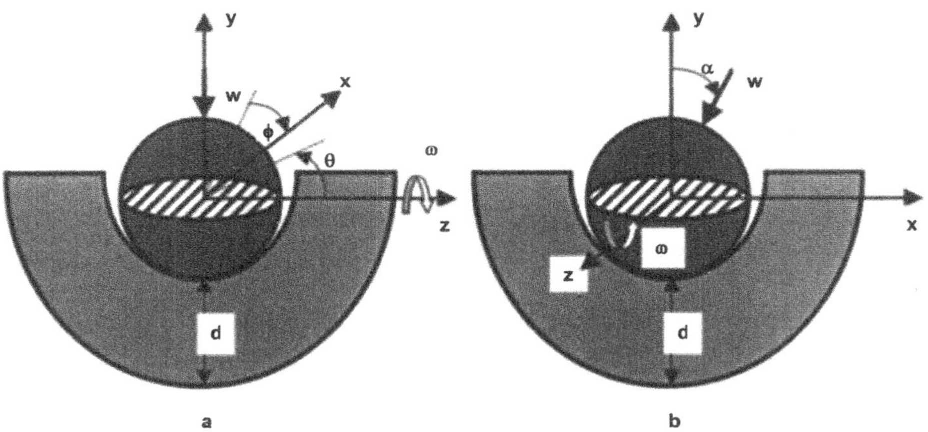

Fig. 6.1 A ball-in-socket model for the elastohydrodynamic lubrication analysis of UHMWPE hip joints

6.3 Governing equations and numerical analysis

The governing equations for the present elastohydrodynamic lubrication problem consist of Reynolds and elasticity equations. The Reynolds equation in a spherical co-ordinate system for the present model shown in Fig. 6.1 is as follows.

$$\sin\theta \frac{\partial}{\partial\theta}\left(h^3 \sin\theta \frac{\partial p}{\partial\theta}\right)+\frac{\partial}{\partial\phi}\left(h^3 \frac{\partial p}{\partial\phi}\right)=6\eta\, R_2^2 \sin^2\theta\left(\omega\frac{\partial h}{\partial\phi}+2\frac{\partial h}{\partial t}\right) \tag{6.1}$$

The elastic deformation of the bearing surfaces is primarily due to the UHMWPE acetabular cup, since the elastic modulus of the femoral head is at least two orders of magnitude greater than that of UHMWPE. Furthermore, the outside of the UHMWPE acetabular cup is usually fixed to a metallic shell or cemented to the bone, which was, therefore, assumed to be rigidly fixed for calculating the elastic deformation. The elastic deformation for the UHMWPE cup was calculated by either the constrained column model or the finite element method. In the case of the constrained column model, the elastic deformation is directly proportional to the local pressure **(8, 9)**

$$\delta=\frac{R_2\left[\left(\frac{R_3}{R_2}\right)^3-1\right]}{E\left[\frac{1}{1-2\upsilon}+\frac{2}{1+\upsilon}\left(\frac{R_3}{R_2}\right)^3\right]}p \tag{6.2}$$

In the case of the finite element model, the UHMWPE cup was meshed into a number of elements (usually 60 × 60 on the bearing surface), and the elastic deformation was obtained by ABAQUS (Version 5.8) **(10)**

$$\delta_{ij}=\sum_{k=1}^{m}\sum_{l=1}^{n}C_{ijkl}\,p_{kl} \tag{6.3}$$

where the displacement coefficients, C_{ijkl} were defined as the average displacement at (i,j) caused by a unit pressure distribution at (k,l).

Other conditions include zero pressure at the edge of the cup and the cavitation boundary whenever the pressure drops to zero, as well as the load balance equation as follows.

$$\begin{aligned}
f_x &= R_2^2\int_0^{\pi}\int_0^{\pi} p\sin\theta\cos\phi\sin\theta\, d\theta\, d\phi = w_x\\
f_y &= R_2^2\int_0^{\pi}\int_0^{\pi} p\sin\theta\sin\phi\sin\theta\, d\theta\, d\phi = w_y\\
f_z &= R_2^2\int_0^{\pi}\int_0^{\pi} p\cos\theta\sin\theta\, d\theta\, d\phi = 0
\end{aligned} \tag{6.4}$$

where w_x and w_y are the resolved components of the applied load (w) in the x and y directions respectively as shown in Fig. 6.1(b). The finite difference method was used to solve both the Reynolds and elasticity equations simultaneously **(10, 11)**.

The transient condition experienced in artificial hip joint replacements during walking requires the solution to both the Reynolds equation including the squeeze-film velocity, and the elasticity equation throughout the walking cycle. This usually takes a significant amount of computing time, and only the column model was used to calculate the elastic deformation. The details of the solution methodology will be reported elsewhere **(12)**.

6.4 Prediction of lubricating film thickness

A typical UHMWPE hip joint replacement was chosen for both steady-state and transient elastohydrodynamic lubrication analyses. The input parameters used for the steady-state analysis are given in Table 6.1.

Table 6.1 Input parameters used for the steady-state elastohydrodynamic lubrication analysis

Femoral head radius (mm)	14
Radial clearance (mm)	0.05* to 0.10
UHMWPE elastic modulus (MPa)	1000
UHMWPE thickness (mm)	7
Poisson's ratio	0.4
Viscosity (Pa s)	0.005 to 1*
Average load (N)	1000* to 2500
Average angular velocity (rad s^{-1})	2

* These values were unrealistic, but chosen to facilitate the convergence of the numerical solutions

6.4.1 Model evaluation under steady-state conditions

6.4.1.1 Comparison between ball-in-socket and ball-on-plane models

A representative viscosity of 0.01 Pa s and load of 2500 N were chosen for this analysis. The simple estimation of the lubricating film thickness for artificial hip joint replacements can be made by using the well-established formulae available in the tribology literature based upon an equivalent ball-on-plane configuration (Fig. 6.2). Such an analysis has been carried out for various forms of artificial hip joint replacements using the well-known Hamrock and Dowson formulae for a sphere on a semi-infinite solid [Fig. 6.2(a)], and an iso-viscous and incompressible fluid **(3)**. However, a more accurate film thickness was predicted based on a layered surface when the contact dimension becomes comparable to the UHMWPE thickness, the assumption of semi-infinite solid is no longer valid and the elastohydrodynamic lubrication for a layered surface as shown in Fig. 6.2(b) is required. Under this latter condition, the film thickness formula obtained by Wang **(13)** based on the constrained column model or by Jin **(14)** based on the full elasticity equation were used to predict the minimum film thickness. Figure 6.3 compares the minimum film thickness predicted from the various models.

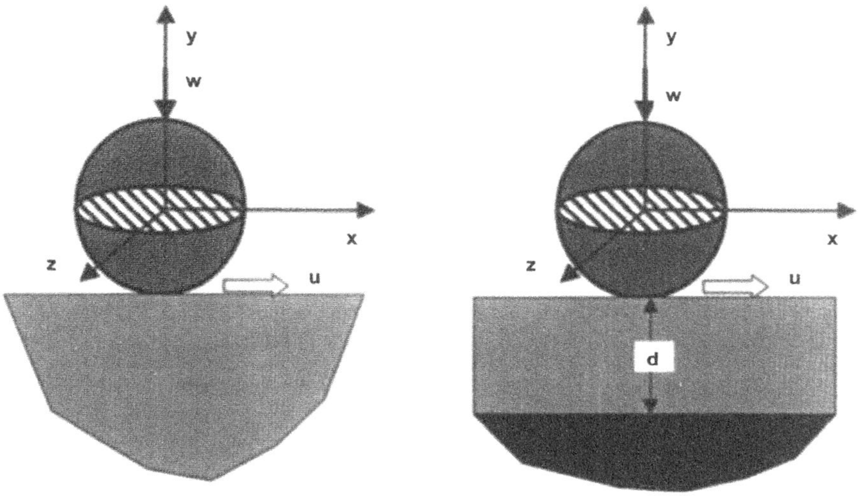

Fig. 6.2 Equivalent ball-on-plane models for the elastohydrodynamic lubrication analysis (a) semi-infinite solid (b) layered surface

It is clear from Fig. 6.3 that the difference in the minimum film thickness predicted is generally very small between all models considered in this study. For example, for the ball-on-plane model, there is little difference in the minimum film thickness predicted between the assumptions of semi-infinite and layered solids, and the use of the column model over-estimates the film thickness by about 25 per cent. The minimum film thickness predicted is decreased by about 10 per cent when the curvature associated with the ball-in-socket model is considered, which is consistent with our previous study **(15)**.

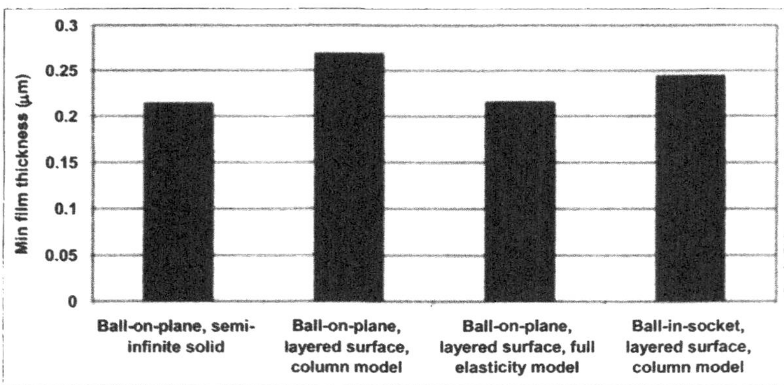

Fig. 6.3 Comparison of the minimum film thickness predicted by different models under steady-state conditions

6.4.1.2 Comparison between the constrained column model and finite element model

A high viscosity of 1 Pa s was chosen for this case in order to obtain convergent solutions from the numerical method incorporating the full elasticity model based on the finite element method for the ball-in-socket configuration. Figure 6.4 shows the comparison of the predicted pressure distributions and the film profiles along the centre line in the entraining direction for both the column model and the finite element model. Little difference can be seen between the two elasticity models in predicting both the pressure distribution and the film profile under elastohydrodynamic lubrication conditions.

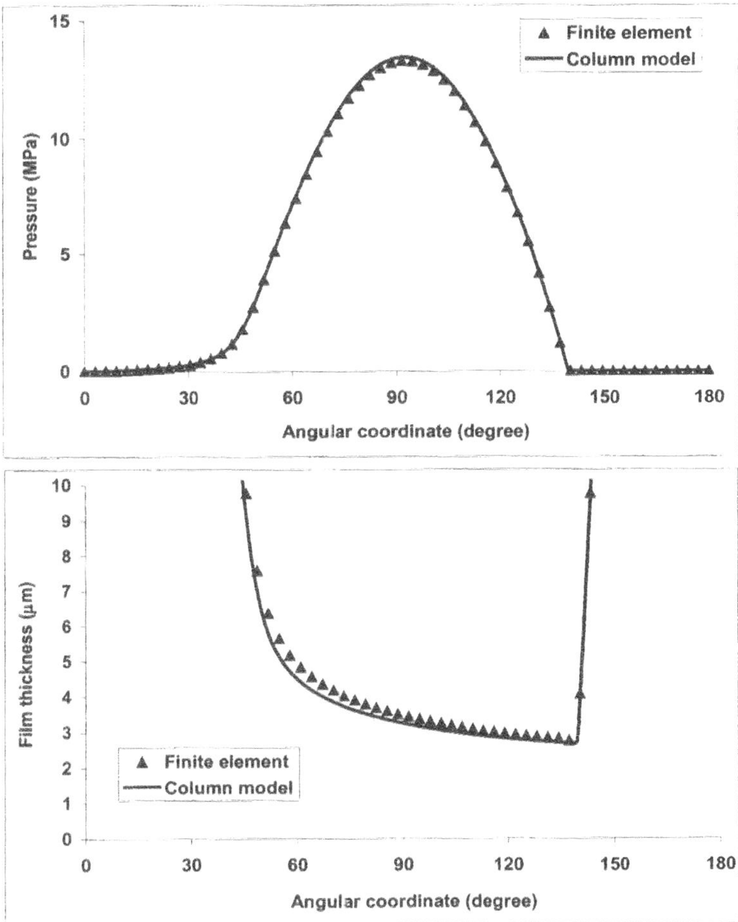

Fig. 6.4 Comparison of the pressure distribution and film thickness predicted by the column and the finite element models for the ball-in-socket configuration

6.4.1.3 Loading direction

A small radial clearance of 0.05 mm and a relatively small load of 1000 N were chosen to investigate the effect of the load angle (α) on the predicted pressure distributions and film profiles as shown in Fig. 6.5, based on the column model.

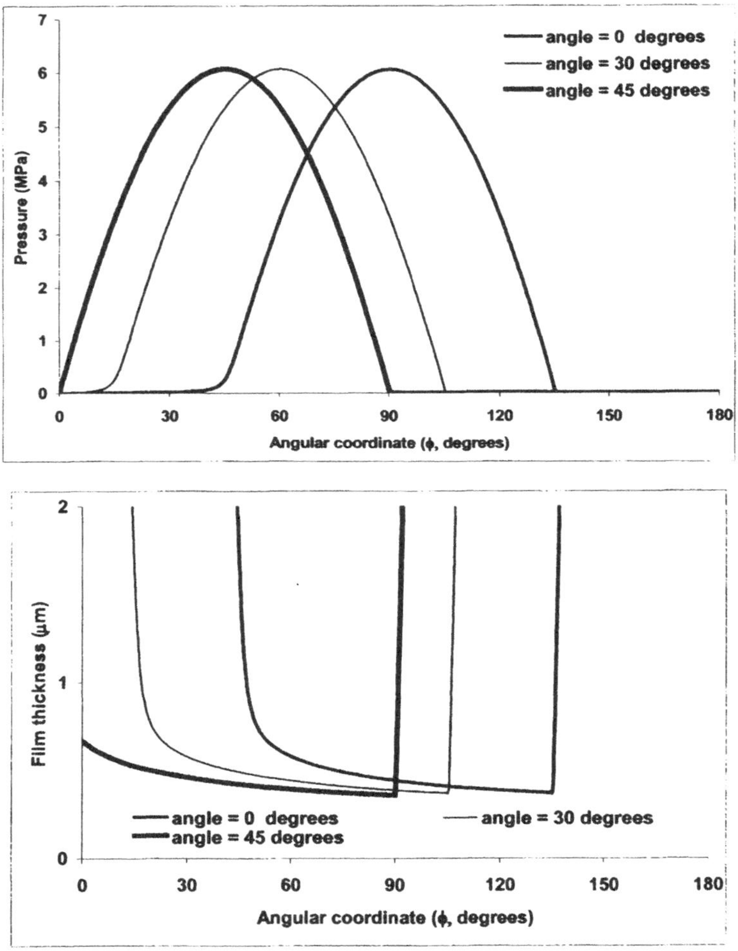

Fig. 6.5 Effect of load angle on the pressure distribution and film thickness predicted by the column model for the ball-in-socket geometry

The change of the load angle from 0 to 45 degrees shifts the contact conjunction to the left of the acetabular cup (Fig. 6.1), and consequently both the pressure distribution and the film profile are closer to the inlet region. There is little difference in the predicted pressure distribution, and the film thickness is only slightly reduced due to the reduction in the inlet region and the lack of pressure build-up. However, this conclusion may not be true if the contact conjunction moves beyond the edge of the cup, and under this condition the film thickness can be expected to decrease dramatically.

6.4.2 Model evaluation under transient conditions

The radial clearance and the viscosity for the transient analysis were chosen as 0.1 mm and 0.01 Pa s respectively, and only the column model was considered for calculating the elastic deformation for this case. Two representative transient conditions were considered, the first case being a variable angular velocity shown in Fig. 6.6(a) and a constant load of 2500 N and the second being a variable load shown in Fig. 6.6(b) and a constant angular velocity of 2 rad s^{-1}. Figures 6.7(a) and 6.7(b) show the predictions of the transient minimum and maximum values of the minimum film thickness through one cycle for the dynamic conditions shown in Figs 6.6(a) and 6.6(b) respectively. The steady-state average values of the minimum film thickness shown in Figs 6.7(a) and 6.7(b) were based upon an average angular velocity of 1 rad s^{-1} and a load of 500 N respectively.

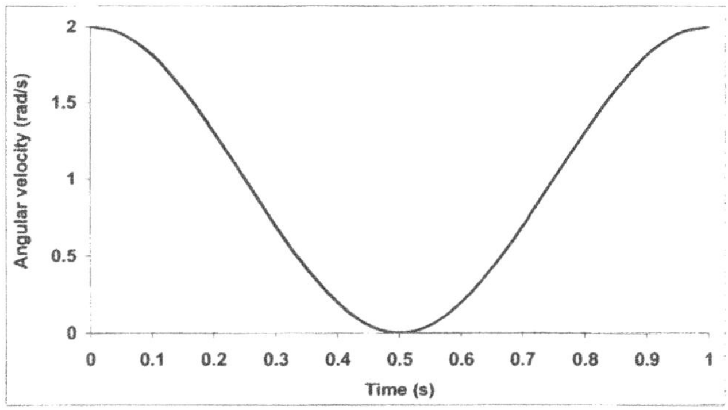

Fig. 6.6(a) Variation of angular velocity used in the transient elastohydrodynamic lubrication analysis under a constant load

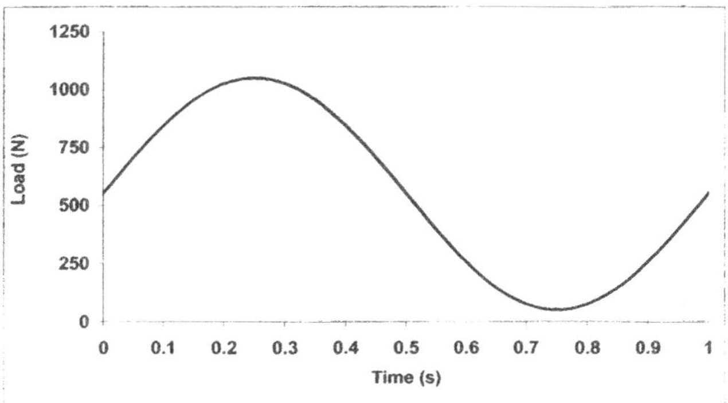

Fig. 6.6(b) Variation of load used in the transient elastohydrodynamic lubrication analysis under a constant angular velocity

The predicted cyclic film thickness for the transient loading conditions shown in Figs 6.6(a) and 6.6(b) is remarkably constant, with a small difference between the minimum and the maximum values as shown in Figs 6.7(a) and 6.7(b). This is consistent with the previous findings that the combined action of entraining and squeeze-film motions maintains a relatively constant lubricating film thickness in synovial joints during steady-state walking **(16)**. Furthermore, it is interesting to note that the average transient minimum film thickness predicted through one simulated cycle is very close to the value based upon average conditions.

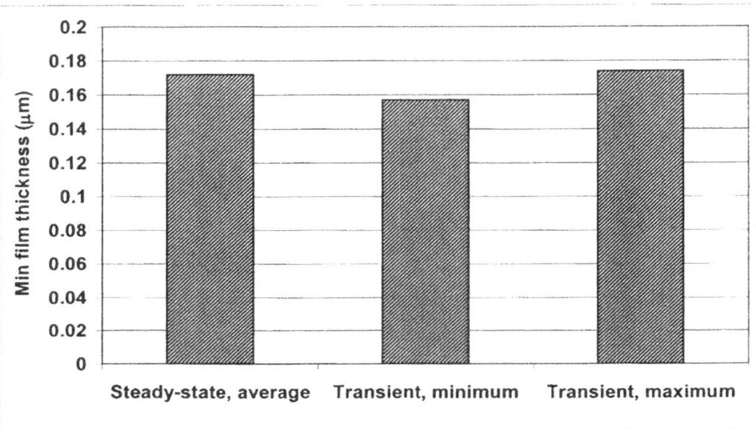

Fig. 6.7(a) Comparison of the minimum film thickness predicted by steady-state and transient analysis for conditions shown in Fig. 6.6(a)

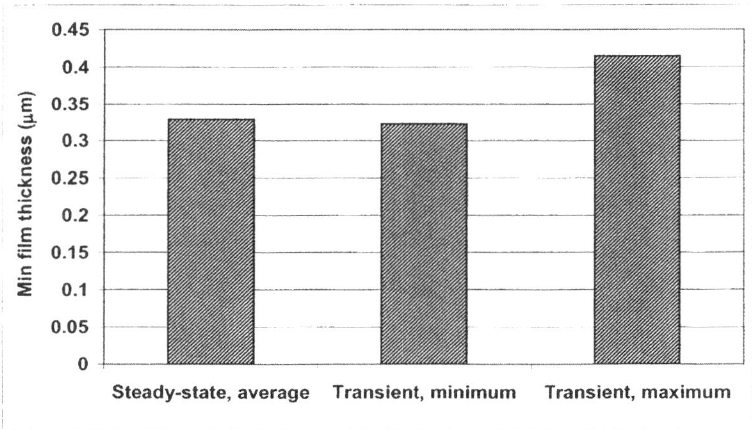

Fig. 6.7(b) Comparison of the minimum film thickness predicted by steady-state and transient analysis for conditions shown in Fig. 6.6(b)

6.4.3 Prediction of the minimum film thickness under more physiological conditions

Some of the parameters for the analyses presented in Sections 6.4.1 and 6.4.2 were primarily chosen to facilitate the numerical solution, and are not representative of more realistic physiological conditions experienced in hip joints during walking. The following parameters were selected to estimate the minimum film thickness likely to be generated in UHMWPE hip joints during steady-state walking:

- viscosity of synovial fluid after total joint replacements 0.005 Pa s
- average angular velocity 1 rad s^{-1}

Under these conditions, the minimum film thickness was predicted to be 0.12 μm. Although the minimum film thickness predicted also depends on the design parameters, the magnitude of the film thickness predicted is generally between 0.1 and 0.25 μm **(15)**. It is clear that the minimum film thickness predicted is much smaller than the surface roughness of the UHMWPE bearing surface, often quoted as between 0.5 and 1 μm **(3)**. Therefore, the present theoretical study confirms the previous experimental findings of a mixed/boundary lubrication regime in UHMWPE hip joint replacements **(2)**.

6.5 Overall discussion and conclusions

It is clear from Section 6.4 that the difference in the minimum film thickness predicted from various models considered in this study is relatively small. The column model is reasonably accurate for the elastic deformation calculation and the corresponding elastohydrodynamic lubrication analysis for UHMWPE hip joints. The remarkably constant film thickness predicted under the transient condition not only makes it possible to estimate the average transient film thickness from the quasi-static steady-state solution using average load and speed, but also suggests that the detailed variation of the load and speed experienced during the hip joint may not be important. The effect of the loading angle has only a small effect on the predicted pressure distribution and the film thickness, provided that the contact conjunction is located within the acetabular cup. Therefore, it can be concluded that the steady-state elastohydrodynamic lubrication analysis based on the column model can be applied to UHMWPE hip joints under physiological conditions.

However, it should be noted that the minimum film thickness predicted for UHMWPE hip joints under physiological conditions is much smaller than the original roughness of the UHMWPE bearing surface, often quoted as 0.5 to 1 μm **(3)**. Therefore, the assumption of smooth bearing surfaces is no longer valid in the elastohydrodynamic lubrication analysis of UHMWPE hip joint replacements. The present analysis can only provide an indication of the severity of the asperity contact and consequently wear. Furthermore, the design parameters should be chosen to minimize wear, rather than the lubricating film thickness if the resultant lubrication is still in the mixed regime. For example, although an increase in the femoral head radius increases both the equivalent radius and the sliding velocity, and consequently the lubricating film thickness, the sliding distance is also increased which may adversely increase the wear.

Despite all these limitations, there are many potential applications of the present lubrication methodology for artificial hip joints in optimizing the tribological performance of these man-made bearings. For example, it is possible to investigate the effect of modification of the radial clearance between the ball and the cup associated with the running-in process as well as the use of cross-linked polyethylene cups where no wear has been observed in simulator studies (**17**). The lubrication methodology can be expected to extend to other forms of bearing couples where fluid-film lubrication may be more important, such as metal-on-metal and ceramic-on-ceramic (**10, 18, 19**).

6.6 Acknowledgement

This work was supported by the Engineering and Physical Sciences Research Council (EPSRC).

References

(1) **Ingham, E.** and **Fisher, J.** Biological reactions to wear debris in total joint replacement, Proc Instn Mech Engr, Journal of Engineering in Medicine, 2000, 214(H1), 21–37.

(2) **Unsworth, A., Dowson, D.**, and **Wright, V.** The frictional behaviour of human synovial joints – Part II. Artificial joints. Trans ASME, Journal of Lubrication Technology, 1975, 97(3), 377–382.

(3) **Jin, Z. M., Dowson, D.**, and **Fisher, J.** Analysis of fluid film lubrication in artificial hip joint replacements with surfaces of high elastic modulus, Proc Instn Mech Engr, Journal of Engineering in Medicine, 1997. 211, 247–256.

(4) **Paul, J. P.** Forces transmitted by joints in the human body, in Lubrication and Wear in Living and Artificial Human Joints, Proc Instn Mech Engr, 1967, 181(3J), 8–15.

(5) **Saarri, H., Santavirta, S., Nordstrom, D., Paavolainen, P.**, and **Konttinen, Y. T.**, Hyaluronate in total hip replacement. J. Rheumatol, 1993, 20(1), 87–90.

(6) **Delecrin, J., Oka, M., Takahashi, S., Yamamuro, T.**, and **Nakamura, T.** Changes in joint fluid after total arthroplasty, clinical orthopaedics and related research, 1994, 307, 240–249.

(7) **Cooke, A. V., Dowson, D.**, and **Wright, V.** The rheology of synovial fluid and some potential synthetic lubricants for degenerate synovial joints. Engng in Medicine, 1978, 7, 66–72.

(8) **Jin, Z. M., Heng, S. M., Ng, H. W.**, and **Auger, D. D.** An axisymmetric contact model of ultra high molecular weight polyethylene cups against metallic femoral heads for artificial hip joint replacements, Proc Instn Mech Engr, Journal of Engineering in Medicine, 1999, 213(H4), 317–327.

(9) **Bartel, D. L., Burstein, A. H., Toda, M. D.**, and **Edwards D. L.** The effect of conformity and plastic thickness on contact stresses in metal-backed plastic implants, Trans ASME, J Biomech Eng, 1985, 107,193–199.

(10) **Jalali-Vahid, D., Jagatia, M., Jin, Z. M.**, and **Dowson, D.** Elastohydrodynamic lubrication analysis of UHMWPE hip joint replacements, in thinning films and tribological interfaces, 26th Leeds-Lyon Symp on Tribology, 2000, 329–339.

(11) **Jagatia, M.** and **Jin, Z. M.** Elastohydrodynamic lubrication analysis of metal-on-metal hip prosthesis under steady-state entraining motion, Proc Instn Mech Engr, Journal of Engineering in Medicine, 2001, submitted.

(12) **Jalali-Vahid, D.** and **Jin, Z. M.** Transient elastohydrodynamic lubrication analysis of UHMWPE hip joint replacements, Proc Instn Mech Engr, Journal of Mechanical Engineering Science, 2002, in press.

(13) **Wang, D.** Elastohydrodynamic lubrication of point contacts for layers of 'soft' solids and monolithic 'hard' materials in the transient bouncing ball problem, 1994, PhD Thesis, University of Leeds, England.

(14) **Jin, Z. M.** Elastohydrodynamic lubrication of circular point contact for a compliant layered surface bonded to a rigid substrate – Part 2 numerical results, Journal of Engineering Tribology, Proc Instn Mech Engr, 2000, 214, 281–289.

(15) **Jalali-Vahid, D., Jagatia, M., Jin, Z. M.,** and **Dowson, D.** Prediction of lubricating film thickness in UHMWPE hip joint replacements, Journal of Biomechanics, 2001, 34, 261–266.

(16) **Jin, Z. M., Dowson, D.,** and **Fisher, J.** Fluid film lubrication in natural hip joints in Thin Films in Tribology (Eds D. Dowson, C. M. Taylor, and M. Godet, Elsevier, Amsterdam), 1993, 545–555.

(17) **Jasty, M., Bragdon, C. R., O'Connor, D. O., Muratoglu, O. K., Premnath, V.,** and **Merrill, E.** Marked improvement in the wear resistance of a new form of uhmwpe in a physiological hip simulator, World Tribology Congress, 8–12 September 1997, 734.

(18) **Chan, F. W., Bobyn, J. D., Medley, J. B., Krygier, J. J.,** and **Tanzer, M.** The Otto Aufranc Award – Wear and lubrication of metal-on-metal hip implants, Clinical Orthopaedics and Related Research, 1999, 369, 10–24.

(19) **Nevelos, J. E., Ingham, E., Doyle, C., Fisher, J.,** and **Nevelos, A. B.** Analysis of retrieved alumina ceramic components from Mittelmeier total hip prostheses, Biomaterials, 1999, 20(19), 1833–40.

Z M Jin, M Jagatia, and **D Jalali-Vahid**
Department of Mechanical and Medical Engineering, University of Bradford, UK

7

Wear of Ceramic-on-ceramic Hip Prostheses under Micro-separation Simulation Conditions

G M Insley, T Stewart, J Nevelos, J Fisher, and **R M Streicher**

Abstract

Standard simulator kinematics are not sufficient to reproduce the wear rates and mechanisms of alumina ceramic hip prostheses which are found in the clinical situation. However, simulation of a micro-separation between the femoral head and acetabular cup during the swing phase in the hip joint simulator has reproduced clinically relevant wear rates, wear patterns, wear mechanisms, and wear debris for alumina/alumina bearings.

7.1 Introduction

The majority of total hip prostheses currently implanted consist of a metal femoral head i.e. (cobalt chrome, nitrogen-strengthened stainless steel) articulating against an ultra-high molecular weight polyethylene (UHMWPE) acetabular cup. Typical wear rates of 40–100 mm^3 per year have been reported corresponding to a linear penetration rate of the femoral head into the acetabular component of less than 0.25 mm per year **(1)**. Even though the majority of these implants are successful there is a growing volume of evidence showing that wear debris from this combination leads to the eventual failure of the prosthesis **(2, 3)**. It is generally believed that UHMWPE wear debris generated at the articulating surface enters the periprosthetic tissue where it triggers a number of defence mechanisms in the bone cells. The end result is osteoclastic bone resorption, leading to osteolysis and eventual loosening of the prosthesis. It is not the volume of wear particles that is important in this mechanism but the number of particles and their size range. Research has shown that particles in the size range 0.2–0.8 μm cause the highest biological response in the body **(1)**.

The growing need to treat younger, more active patients has led to alternative bearing materials. Examples are the hard-on-hard bearing combinations of ceramic-on-ceramic and metal-on-metal. Ceramic-on-ceramic replacement hip joints have been in use since 1970. The earliest examples of ceramic-on-ceramic total hip replacements and surface replacements were those designed by Boutin, Griss, Salzer, and Mittelmeier. These involved alumina femoral heads articulating against alumina acetabular cups, and were designed to provide low wear and good durability. Alumina ceramics are compounds in their highest oxidation state, making them chemically inert. Additionally ceramics are very hard (alumina has a Vickers hardness of 1900 kgf mm^{-2}), and are also hydrophilic which means that the surfaces have very good wettability. Furthermore, it is possible to polish ceramics to a very smooth finish with surface roughnesses (R_a) of <0.005 μm. These factors combine to give ceramic counterfaces excellent tribological properties with potential for fluid-film lubrication during walking **(4)**. The wettability and the smoothness of the ceramic surfaces aids in this lubrication, while the hardness and low friction of the surfaces resist damage and wear.

Wear rates of early alumina-on-alumina hip prostheses manufactured from first generation alumina have been shown to be low *in vivo*, ranging from 1 to 5 mm^3 per year **(5)**. The vast majority of retrieved components showed similar characteristic features within the worn bearing surfaces. These included:

- an elliptical wear stripe on the head with maximum penetration up to 100 μm;
- a worn area in the cup with evidence of rim wear;
- an intergranular fracture wear mechanism.

Characteristically these early prostheses were revised for loosening of the acetabular cups, which was partly attributed to the poor fixation of the acetabular component to the bone.

In contrast, simulator testing of ceramic-on-ceramic hip prostheses yielded extremely low wear rates (<0.1mm^3 per million cycles), an order of magnitude lower than those reported *in vivo*. Bearing surfaces were undamaged, with no noticeable change in surface roughness **(6)**.

The wear stripes found in first generation alumina ceramics were believed to be related to the inferior quality of the ceramic material. Developments such as hot isostatic pressing (HIPing) and grain refinement, to increase the density and strength of the alumina, were considered to alleviate this problem. However, recently two modern alumina-on-alumina hip prostheses manufactured from second generation HIPed alumina retrieved after only one year showed wear patterns similar to those found in the early retrieved components, with a small elliptical wear stripe on the femoral head 2–5 μm deep and a small amount of wear on the rim of the acetabular cup. These two prostheses (Fig. 7.1) were both revised due to trauma and were anatomically positioned and well fixed prior to revision **(7)**. Wear volumes for these components have been measured to be approximately 0.5 mm^3.

Wear patterns and mechanisms found clinically were not replicated in standard *in vitro* simulator tests.

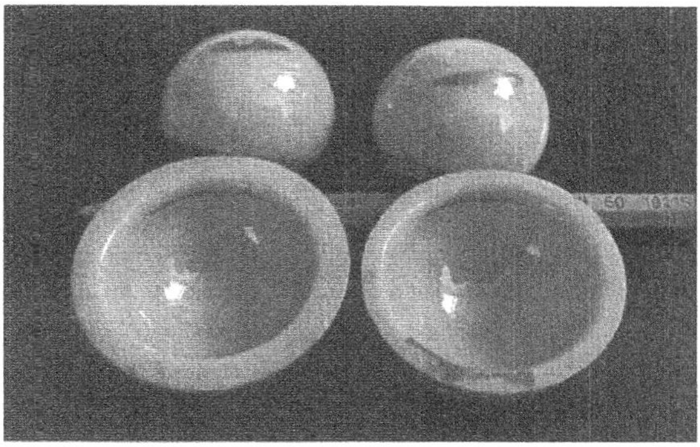

Fig. 7.1 Wear stripes on explanted HIPed alumina-on-alumina components after one year *in vivo* – the wear on the head and insert has been emphasized by rubbing with a graphite pencil

Mallory *et al.* **(8)** found by examining the fluoroscopic images of ten patients walking on a treadmill that the head and cup separate by a small amount during the swing phase. They found that the maximum separation was 2.8 mm and the minimum was 0.8 mm with an average separation seen at 1.2 mm. They also found that while the femoral head separated from the cup it remained in contact with the rim and postulated that high contact stresses would occur at this point with the application of load at heel-strike.

From this research it was hypothesized that micro-separation of the head and cup could occur with any joint replacement and that this could be a factor in wear initiation for ceramic-on-ceramic systems as seen *in vivo*. Typically with these systems there is a very small clearance between the head and cup, of the order of 40 μm, and it is these tight clearances that allow the femoral head to contact the rim of the cup with only limited translation (Fig. 7.2). Contact would occur with lateral and inferior displacements of less than 1 mm for a well-positioned prosthesis. Upon heel-strike the head will translate superiorly and contact the rim before relocating. This rim contact will occur under very high stress and may initiate surface damage and hence accelerate wear **(7)**.

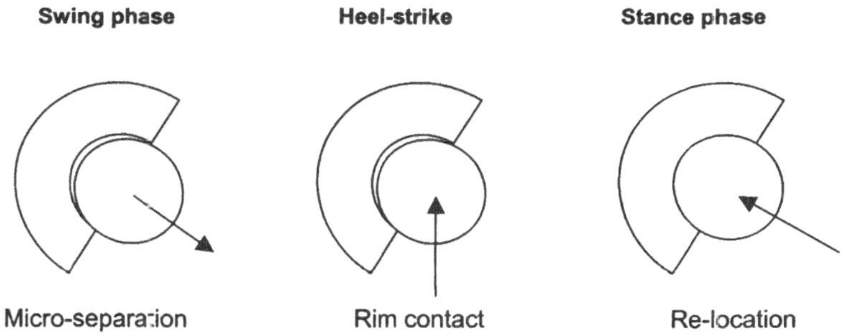

Fig. 7.2 Schematic diagram showing the stages of micro-separation during the walking cycle

This Chapter describes the wear of current and future ceramic-on-ceramic bearing couples under micro-separation conditions in a laboratory simulator.

7.2 Micro-separation

In vitro micro-separation was first reproduced by Nevelos *et al.* (2000) using the Leeds Mk II physiological hip joint simulator **(7)**. Under standard conditions this simulator applied a small positive swing phase load that ensured that the head remained located correctly in the cup throughout the gait cycle. To achieve joint separation a small lateral to medial load was applied to the acetabular insert, which, during the swing phase when the joint load was reduced, produced medial and superior translation of the insert relative to the head. Joint separation was limited by the radial clearance between the articulating components and ceased when the superior rim of the insert contacted the head after approximately 0.5 mm of translation. Further impact of the head and cup occurred with reapplication of the joint load at heel-strike. The load was momentarily supported by the small contact at the rim before the head relocated in the insert, thus modelling the clinical observations shown in Fig. 7.2.

The micro-separation technique reproduced for the first time clinically relevant levels of wear in ceramic-on-ceramic hip prostheses. The technique produced stripe wear with alumina-on-alumina via a similar intergranular fracture wear mechanism (Fig. 7.3) to that seen *in vivo*. For additional validation of the technique, debris collected from the simulator were compared to debris from retrieved tissues; both were found to contain predominantly nanometer-sized ceramic debris with the addition of a few larger ceramic particles attributed to micro-separation.

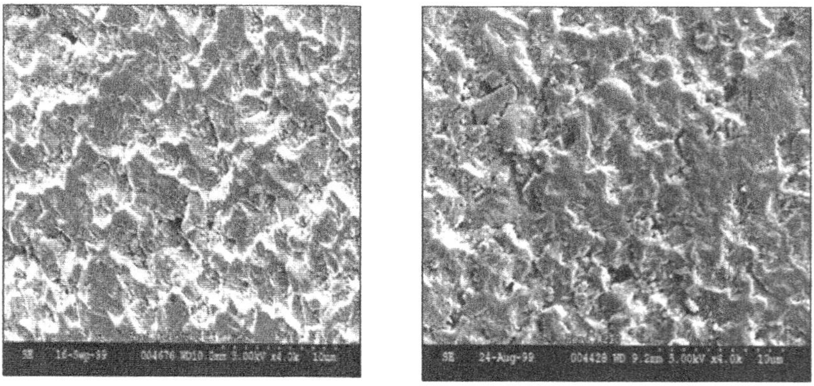

Fig. 7.3 SEM of retrieved (left) and *in vitro* micro-separation (right) head wear stripes

Further research by Stewart *et al.* (2001) showed that when the swing phase load in the simulator was reduced it becomes easier for the medial separation force both to overcome friction and to produce superior translation between the head and insert **(9)**. This increased the velocity of the insert and upon impact of the insert and head produced an increased momentum and impact energy, which resulted in a more severe micro-separation condition. Therefore, by decreasing the swing phase load greater levels of joint laxity were modelled.

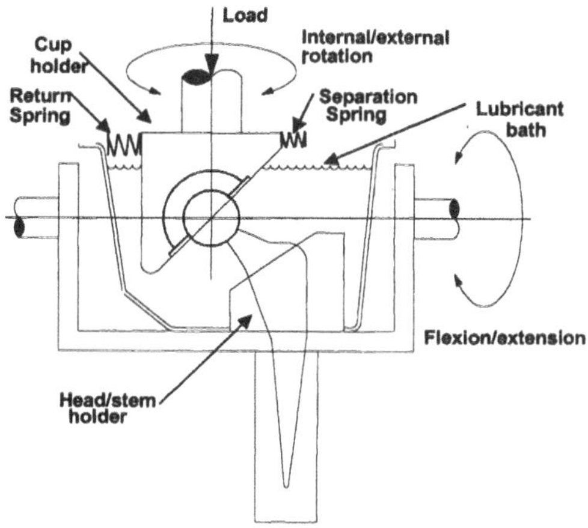

Fig. 7.4 Schematic diagram of the Leeds Mk II physiological hip joint simulator with micro-separation

7.3 Ceramics for hip prostheses

Alumina ceramic has been improved over the past 30 years and the introduction of hot isostatic pressing and grain refinement resulted in improved material properties, as shown in Table 7.1 **(10)**.

Table 7.1 Ceramic materials for hip prostheses

Ceramic	*First generation alumina*	*Third generation alumina*	*Zirconia toughened alumina*
Grain size (μm)	<10	<2	<2
Flexural strength (MPa)	400	580	1150
Density (Mg m^{-3})	3.95	3.98	4.36
Hardness (HV)		2300	1975
Fracture toughness (MPa $m^{1/2}$)		4.3	8.5
Roughness R_a (μm)	<0.05	<0.005	<0.005

One of the main disadvantages of ceramics in joint replacement has been their brittleness. Although the current reported fracture rate is low, typically 1 in 25000 **(9)**, this remains a concern for some surgeons.

The addition of ~25 wt. per cent zirconia to the alumina matrix during manufacture has been shown to increase the fracture toughness and flexural strength of the alumina **(10, 11, 12)**. Two zirconia-toughened aluminas (ZTAs) are currently available, one containing 74 wt. per cent alumina, 24 wt. per cent zirconia, and 1 per cent mixed oxides, and another consisting of 75 wt. per cent alumina and 25 wt. per cent zirconia.

7.4 Ceramic wear

The volumetric wear from standard simulator testing of alumina ceramic-on-ceramic bearings has generally been reported as <0.1 mm³ per million cycles. Micro-separation simulation has been shown to increase this by a factor of ten, approaching clinical levels of wear as seen in retrieved first generation alumina hip prostheses (Fig. 7.5).

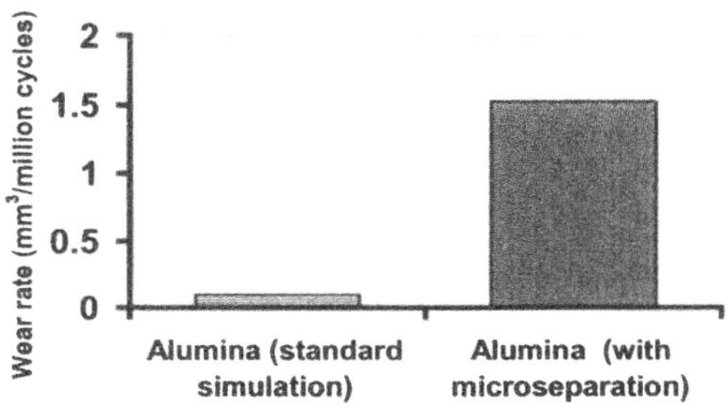

Fig. 7.5 *In vitro* ceramic wear – comparison of standard and micro-separation simulator tests [7]

Micro-separation simulator studies have only, as yet, been reported from one centre. The findings so far support its use as a means to evaluate ceramic bearing materials in a more physiologically realistic manner.

Long term testing has been reported for the current generation of alumina hip prostheses **(9)** with typical wear behaviour as shown in Fig. 7.6.

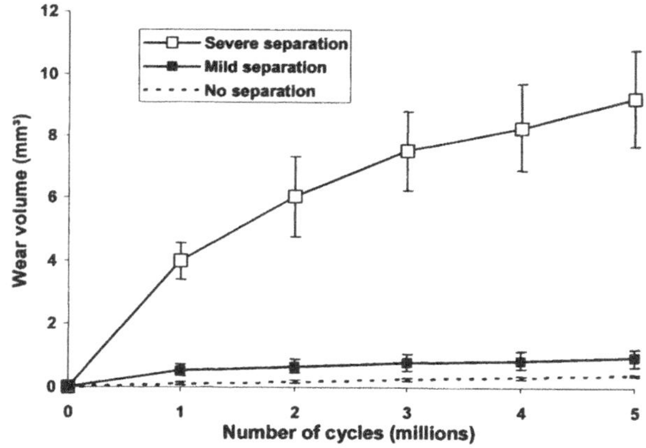

Fig. 7.6 Wear volumes ± standard error, n = 3 for each group

For the current alumina materials under severe micro-separation, wear was characterized by an initially higher wear period during which a characteristic wear stripe on the femoral head and the rim wear on the cup were initiated. The wear then decreased to a lower steady-state value with no signs of run-away wear observed. The severity of testing made a significant difference to the resulting wear rates of the alumina material, emphasizing the need for careful control of experiments.

Worn surfaces appeared as shown in Fig. 7.7, in which the wear on the head and insert has been emphasized by rubbing with a graphite pencil.

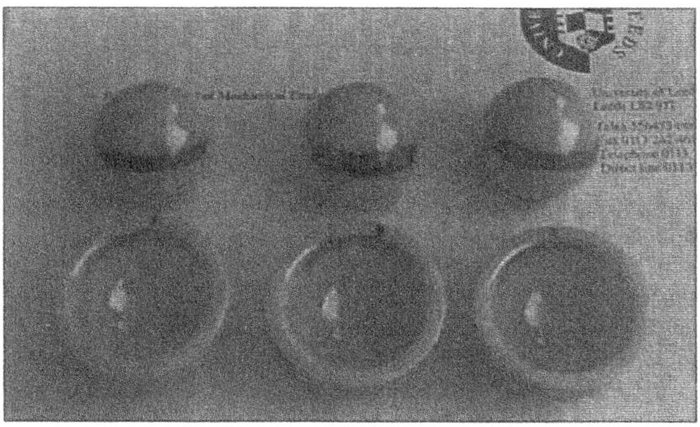

Fig. 7.7 Wear stripes on the alumina-on-alumina components after five million cycles in the Leeds hip simulator under micro-separation conditions

Scanning electron microscopy (SEM) was used to examine the wear scars at a microscopic level. The scars produced by micro-separation testing were remarkably similar to the wear scars seen on the explanted ceramics (Fig. 7.3) and a similar grain boundary fracture wear mechanism was observed.

Wear debris collected and analysed from micro-separation simulation of alumina-on-alumina were generally very small with a mean particle size of approximately 40 nm, as shown in Fig. 7.8. This was similar to the debris collected from normal simulator tests with a mean particle size of 30 nm. The size range of these particles showed that the micro-separation debris also contains a few larger particles that are not seen in normal simulation. Typically these were in the range of 100–3000 nm and compare well to the larger particles seen in the surrounding tissue of retrieved ceramic components.

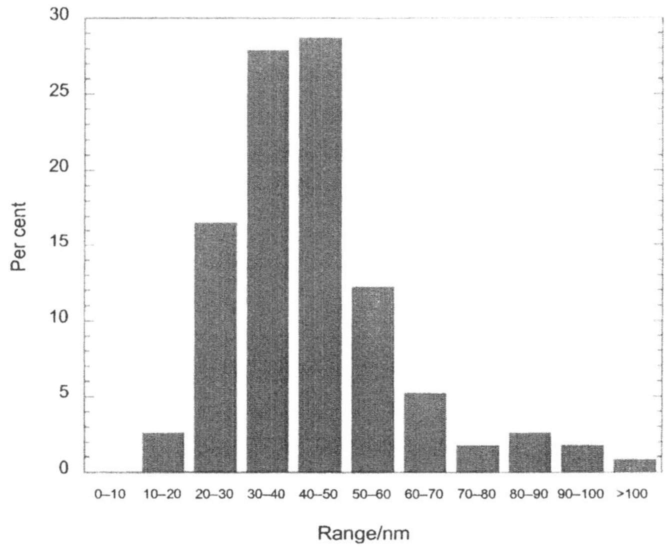

Fig. 7.8 Particle size distribution for wear debris from HIPed alumina tested in the simulator under micro-separation conditions

Preliminary simulator studies have also been completed for two different ZTA materials under standard and micro-separation conditions with the results shown in Fig. 7.9. The materials were tested in a concurrent study with HIPed alumina as a control, for a duration of one million cycles.

Under normal simulation conditions both ZTA materials showed slightly less wear than alumina-on-alumina. Under micro-separation mode, the wear for all couples increased. However, the ZTA-on-ZTA couples wore less than the equivalent alumina-on-alumina couple.

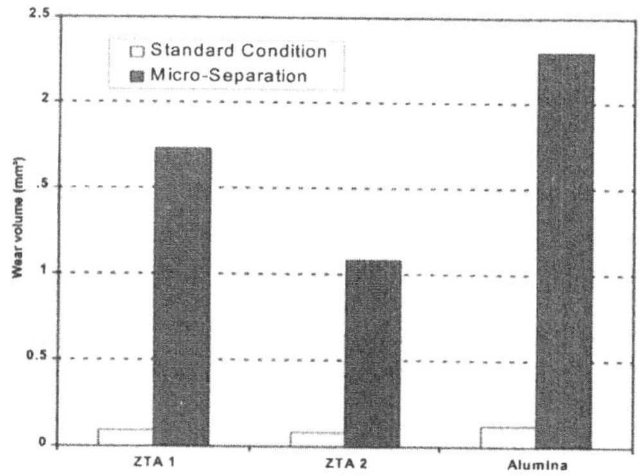

Fig. 7.9 Wear volume of two ZTA materials in standard and micro-separation simulator testing conditions compared to alumina

7.5 Conclusions

Standard simulator kinematics are not sufficient to reproduce the wear rates and mechanisms of alumina ceramic hip prostheses which are found in the clinical situation. However, simulation of a micro-separation between the femoral head and acetabular cup during the swing phase in the hip joint simulator has reproduced clinically relevant wear rates, wear patterns, wear mechanisms, and wear debris for alumina-on-alumina bearings.

Despite the increase in wear volume produced by the micro-separation of ceramic-on-ceramic bearings the wear still remains significantly lower than the wear of traditional metal on UHMWPE bearings.

Preliminary results using zirconia toughened alumina composite ceramics show slightly lower wear than the alumina-on-alumina couple.

References

(1) **Ingham, E.** and **Fisher, J.** Biological reactions to wear debris in total joint replacement. *Proc. Instn. Mech. Engrs.*, Vol 214 Part H, 2000, 21–37.

(2) **Amstutz, H. C., Campbell, P., Kossovsky, N.,** and **Clarke, I. C.** Mechanism and clinical significance of wear debris induced osteolysis. *Clin. Orthop.*, 1992, 276, 7–18.

(3) **Maloney, W. J., Jasty, M., Rosenberg, A.,** and **Harris, W. H.** Bone lysis in well fixed cemented femoral components. *J. Bone Jt. Surgery*, 1990, 72B, 966–970.

(4) **Jin, Z. M., Dowson, D.,** and **Fisher, J.** Analysis of fluid film lubrication in artificial hip joint replacements with surfaces of high elastic modulus. *Proc. Instn. Mech. Engrs.*, Vol H 211, 247–256, 1997.

(5) **Nevelos, J. E., Ingham, E., Doyle, C., Fisher, J.,** and **Nevelos, A. B.** Analysis of retrieved alumina ceramic components from Mittelmeier total hip prostheses. *Journal of Biomaterials*, 20, 1833–1840, 2000.

(6) **Fisher, J., Besong, A. A., Firkins, P. J., Barbour, P. S. M., Nevelos, J. E., Tipper, J. L., Stone M. H.,** and **Ingham, E.** Trans 45th Orthopaedic Research Society, *Proceedings of the 6th World Congress of Biomaterials*, 871, 2000.

(7) **Nevelos, J. E., Ingham, E., Doyle, C., Streicher, R., Nevelos, A. B., Walter, W.,** and **Fisher, J.** Microseparation of the centres of Alumina-Alumina artificial hip joints during simulator testing produces clinically relevant wear rates and patterns. *Journal of Arthroplasty*, 15, 793–795, 2000.

(8) **Mallory, T. H., Dennis, D. A., Northcut, E. J., Lombardi Jr., A. V.,** and **Herrington, S. M.** Do total hip arthoplasty piston during leg length maneuvers and Gait? An *in-vivo* determination of total hip athroplasty separation during abduction/adduction leg lift and gait. Scientific Exhibit 66, AAOS, Los Angeles, CA, USA, 1999.

(9) **Stewart, T., Tipper, J., Streicher, R., Ingham, E.,** and **Fisher, J.** Long term wear of HIPed alumina on alumina bearings for THR under microseparation conditions. *Journal of Materials Science*. In Press.

(10) **Rack, R.** and **Pfaff, H. G.** A new ceramic material for orthopaedics. *Proceedings of the 5th International Biolox Symposium*, March 23–24, 141–145 (2000) Published by Thieme.

(11) **Wang, J.** and **Stevens, R.** Zirconia Toughened Alumina (ZTA) ceramics. *Journal of Materials Science*, 24 (1989) 3421–3440.

(12) **Orange, G.** and **Fantozzi, G.** Comportement mecanique de composites ceramiques à dispersoides. Materiaux et Techniques – Mars (1988), 29–39.

G M Insley
Stryker SA, Scientific and Clinical Affairs, Limerick, Ireland
T Stewart, J Nevelos, and **J Fisher**
School of Mechanical Engineering, University of Leeds, UK
R M Streicher
Stryker SA, Scientific and Clinical Affairs, Thalwil, Switzerland

8

Friction and Wear Testing of DLC Type Coatings on Total Hip Replacement Prostheses

A H S Jones, S K Taylor, D G Teer, and **M Elloy**

Abstract

During a research program to develop diamond-like-carbon (DLC) coatings for total hip replacement (THR) prostheses a new type of carbon coating was developed which now has the trade name Graphit-iC™. This coating gave exceptional friction and wear results in simple laboratory tests against metal counterfaces, but not against UHMWPE as originally intended. Attention then focused on the development of a Graphit-iC coated metal-on-metal THR, and laboratory tests predicted a prosthetic lifetime in excess of 50 years. Coatings were subsequently applied to actual prostheses and tested on the University of Leeds physiological hip simulator. Coating failure was detected on some pairs, yet one pair showed no detectable wear. Parallel testing at Leeds in serum using the simple pendulum simulator failed to show any coating failure. The laboratory test results will be presented and discussed, and speculation made on the reasons for coating failure and the test methods used.

8.1 Introduction

The most widely used artificial hip joints consist of a metal femoral ball, and an acetabular cup made from ultra-high molecular weight polyethylene (UHMWPE). The main cause of failure was loosening of the joint attributable to friction but more importantly wear debris from the UHMWPE **(1)**. The worn particles of UHMWPE were causing adverse biological tissue reactions in areas surrounding the joint, resulting in the loss of supporting bone by resorption. In this way the implant loosened and it life limited **(2)**. Increased UHMWPE wear was attributable to third-body damage to the metal ball resulting in accelerated abrasive wear. Attempts to reduce UHMWPE wear include the use of hard, through fragile, ceramic heads and by the use of many types of surface modification to the metal ball, culminating in hard coatings such as TiN.

Due to a combination of low friction, wear resistance, and chemical inertness, DLC coatings were considered ideal for the protection of femoral heads and the reduction of UHMWPE wear. A programme of work was undertaken to improve the friction and wear of UHMWPE sliding on CoCrMo by coating the metal with DLC. However, it was found that a-C:H:Me DLC coatings deposited by a typical plasma assisted CVD technique **(3)** on to CoCrMo actually increased the coefficient of friction when sliding against UHMWPE in water, when compared to the uncoated CoCrMo. There was also no evidence that the DLC had reduced the UHMWPE wear **(4)**. In order to improve the friction and wear characteristics, efforts were made to develop a DLC coating with superior tribological properties. A new DLC coating, now known as Graphit-iC™, was deposited by sputtering carbon targets in a pure argon atmosphere, and was shown to have lower friction, higher wear resistance, and a greater load bearing capacity when tested against metal counterparts **(5, 6)**.

However, when rubbed against the UHMWPE the friction was again found to be significantly higher than for the uncoated metal. Various types of DLC coatings on CoCrMo substrates were obtained from many leading laboratories around the world and were tested against UHMWPE. In all cases the friction was higher than for the uncoated CoCrMo when rubbing against UHMWPE. It was therefore concluded that these DLC coatings were not capable of reducing the friction and wear of the UHMWPE, although the authors acknowledge that Lappalainen *et al.* have since reported a reduction in friction by using polished amorphous diamond coatings **(7)**.

Due to the Graphit-iC coatings' excellent tribological properties, in water as well as air, it was decided to investigate their potential in improving the performance of metal-on-metal THRs. The McKee CoCrMo metal-on-metal THR was introduced in the 1950s, but poor manufacturing tolerances and unsuitable ball-to-cup clearances, resulting in unacceptably high friction, limited the success of metal-on-metal prostheses. Low friction and low initial wear results of the Charnley-type THR made metal against UHMWPE the method of choice, thus curtailing the development of the metal-on-metal joint. Failure of most metal-on-metal joints was attributed to friction but some did survive and, years later, when explanted and examined, the wear was found to be extremely low, in the range 2–20 μm per year, compared to 100–200 μm per year for UHMWPE against metal or ceramic **(8)**. This reduction of wear gave renewed interest to the metal-on-metal type THR and its development has continued to the present day, now with even more vigour **(9)**.

Simple configuration laboratory testing provided specific wear rates of 2×10^{-15} m^3 N^{-1} m^{-1} for high carbon (0.2–0.3 per cent) CoCrMo alloy with friction coefficients μ of ~0.2 in metal pin on metal disc tests lubricated with serum **(10)**. When compared to the specific wear rate of Graphit-iC™ in ambient conditions of 3×10^{-17} m^3 N^{-1} m^{-1} and friction coefficients <0.1 it became apparent that large increases in lifetimes might be obtainable by applying the Graphit-iC™ coating to metal-on-metal hip joints.

Early results of simple wear tests comparing the friction and wear of coated and uncoated metal-on-metal bearings were very promising. Metal-on-metal hip prostheses manufactured by Avatar Medical Limited (now Zynergy Orthopaedics Limited) were coated by TCL and tested at the University of Leeds in a pendulum-type simulator, short term, and long term in the physiological simulator. This Chapter presents the results of both sets of wear testing, analyses the coating performance in terms of wear mechanisms and failure modes, and assesses its future potential in prosthetics.

8.2 Experimental details

The coatings reported here were deposited in a Teer UDP650, four magnetron, sputter ion plating coating system. The deposition details have been published previously **(5, 6, 11)**. Pure carbon films were used in the initial study: these were 1 μm thick. Multi-layered Graphit-iC films produced later were 2.5 μm thick. The initial coating development results were obtained from coatings deposited on M42 grade tool steel. For application to prostheses, coatings were deposited on to samples machined from wrought CoCrMo alloy (Co-27Cr-5.5Mo-0.06C) conforming to ASTM F799-96 and ISO5832 part 12:1996(E). The CoCrMo samples were finished to $R_a < 0.05\mu m$, to be comparable with the finish of actual implants.

Initial tests were performed at Teer Coatings Limited (TCL) on coated M42 tool steel samples, using a uni-directional pin-on-disc tester. Normal loads of up to 100 N were applied to a 5 mm diameter WC-6%Co ball sliding at a speed of 200 mm s^{-1}, in ambient air. Reciprocating wear tests were used to assess the wear of 3 mm diameter flat ended UHMWPE pins (GUR 415HP) after sliding against Graphit-iC coated, and uncoated, CoCrMo flat samples in de-ionized water. These tests were performed at 3 mm s^{-1} constant sliding speed, 0.5 Hz, for a duration of 10 000 cycles. To assess the performance of Graphit-iC coatings on metal-on-metal couples, Graphit-iC coated, and uncoated, 5 mm diameter, hemispherically ended, CoCrMo pins were tested against Graphit-iC coated, and uncoated, flat CoCrMo samples. Normal loads of 5 N and 40 N were used respectively, in de-ionized water or laboratory atmosphere (ambient, 20 °C, 40–60 per cent RH) conditions. Friction was continuously recorded during the tests. Wear of coatings on flat samples was assessed by producing ball craters on wear tracks. This is a simple method which provides a tapered cross section of the coating. An optical microscope can then be used to obtain information such as depth of wear, plastic deformation of both the coating and substrate, and coating–substrate interface condition **(12, 13)**.

Reciprocating wear tests were performed at the University of Leeds to record friction and wear between Graphit-iC coated CoCrMo (low carbon content) pins and flat plates. The pins used were 12 mm diameter, 100 mm radius of curvature of tip with a 3 mm diameter flat. To make friction measurements, 10 and 20 N normal loads were used with a 30 mm track length, 0.5 Hz or 30 mm s^{-1}, with a 25 per cent bovine serum lubricant. Wear tests were then performed at a normal load of 80 N (11.3 MPa), 30 mm wear track length, 1 Hz for a total of four 24-hour periods. The wear was measured by weighing.

Metal-on-metal THRs were manufactured by Avatar Medical Limited from wrought CoCrMo alloy. These had a head diameter of 28 mm and radial clearances varied from 50 μm to 550 μm. A 53 mm diameter pair with a radial clearance of 50 μm was also manufactured. These were then coated with the Graphit-iC coating (Fig. 8.1) at Teer Coatings Limited, and supplied for test.

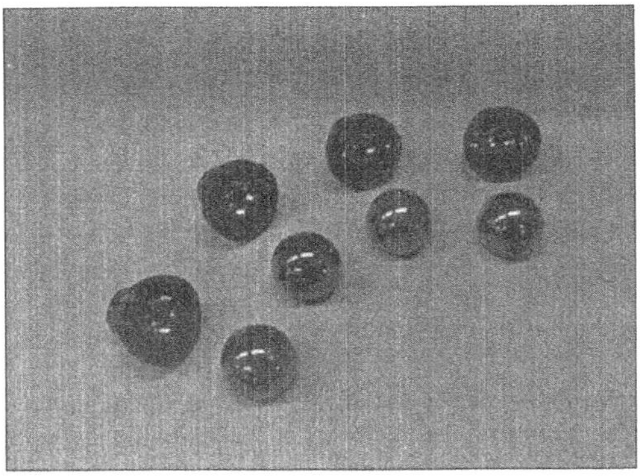

Fig. 8.1 Graphit-iC coated metal-on-metal modular hip prostheses (femoral head diameter 28 mm)

The hip joint couples were used first in a study of friction. Frictional torque was recorded for the different pairings of head and cup at a constant load of 500 N in a driven pendulum friction rig. Each pairing was tested in the presence of water, Ringer's solution, 25 per cent bovine calf serum and with no lubricant (dry). A CoCrMo Metasul pairing was also used as a comparison, plus metal/UHMWPE and alumina/alumina pairs.

The same head and cup pairings were then tested on a physiological simulator which consisted of two articulating stations and one dynamically loaded creep station. The prostheses were mounted in the anatomical position and experienced three directional forces (vertical, anterior–posterior, and medial–lateral) and three degrees of motion (flexion–extension, abduction–adduction, and rotational) as defined by Paul **(14)**. All tests were performed in 25 per cent bovine serum (0.1 per cent sodium azide).

8.3 Results and discussion

The carbon coating, Graphit-iC, was originally developed to give improved performance over conventional hydrogenated DLC in wear applications. This was achieved using conventional wear tests in ambient air, oil, and water against hard counterfaces such as WC or Cr-steel balls. The coatings were found to have good friction characteristics and excellent wear resistance in these situations, as shown in Fig. 8.2(a) and (b). The coatings had a plastic hardness (analogous to Vickers) of around 1600 kg mm^{-2} at a load of 50 mN, and excellent adhesion provided by a Cr interlayer, shown by the Rockwell indent in Fig. 8.2(c). The deposition technique utilizing multiple magnetron sputtering sources allowed the films to be deposited as pure carbon mono-layers, or as carbon/Cr multilayers. These fine multi-layers, or nano-layers can be seen in Fig. 8.3 in a TEM cross section produced at the University of Northumbria.

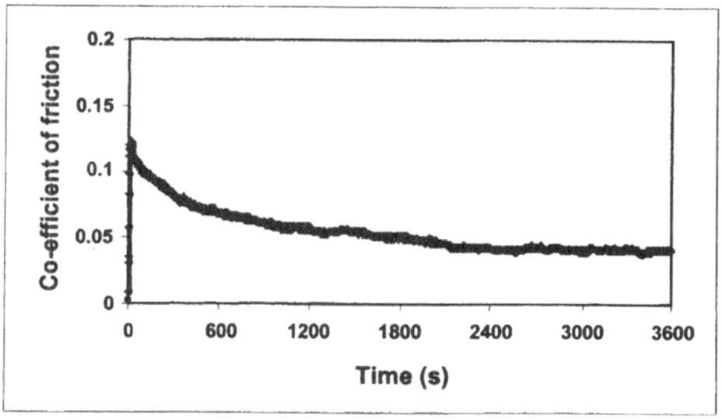

(a) Friction trace during an 80 N uni-directional pin-on-disc test performed in air

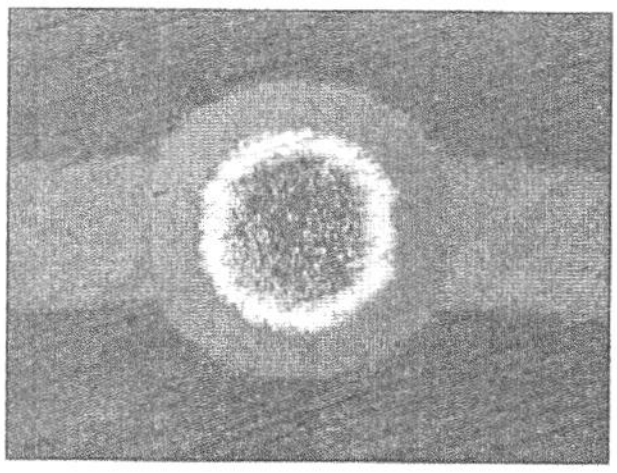

(b) Ball crater on the wear track of the pin-on-disc test shown in (a)

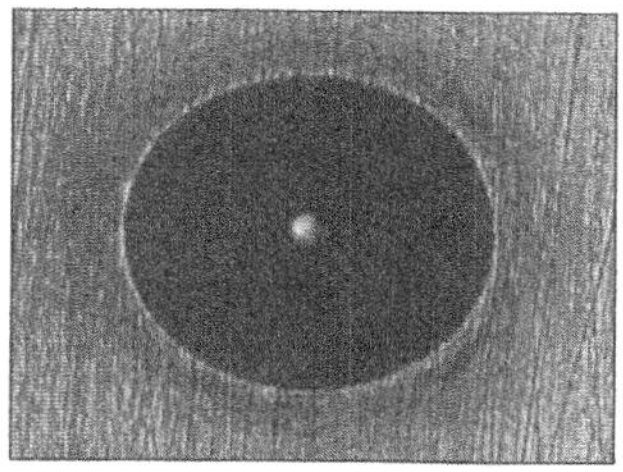

(c) Rockwell C indent used to indicate coating adhesion

Fig. 8.2 Graphit-iC wear characteristics

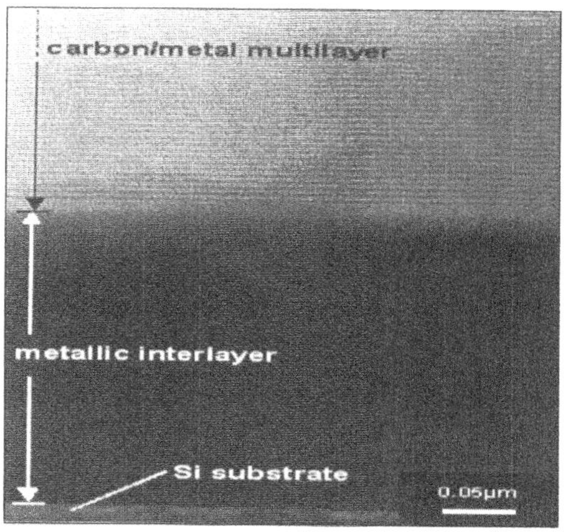

Fig. 8.3 TEM cross section showing the interlayer and the multi-layer structure

When the coating was deposited on to CoCrMo and tested against an UHMWPE pin in deionized water, the friction was higher than that found for uncoated CoCrMo. The difference was at least a factor of two, as seen in Fig. 8.4(a), and it was shown that this was not a result of surface roughness. The low friction of the solid lubricant coatings when sliding against UHMWPE was now brought into question, and therefore a number of DLC coatings from around the world were obtained and tested against UHMWPE. The results are shown in Fig. 8.4(b) where it can be seen that none of the DLC coatings produced the low coefficient of friction of around 0.06 that was obtained against CoCrMo in these short-term tests.

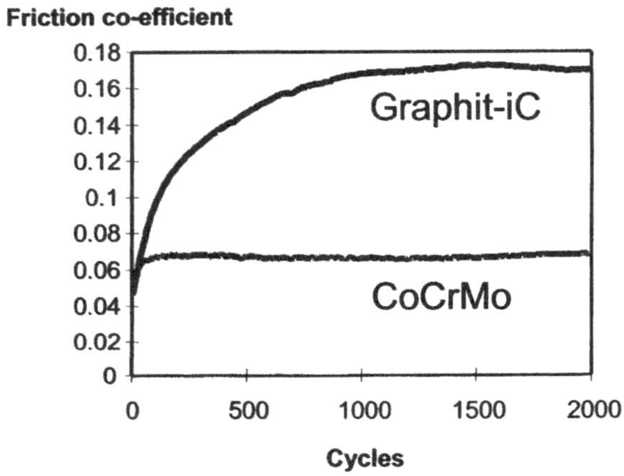

(a) Friction during reciprocating wear test in water of UHMWPE against Graphit-iC and uncoated CoCrMo

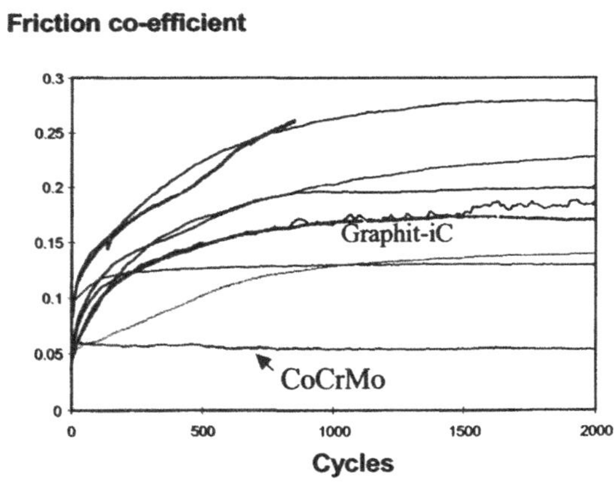

(b) Friction coefficients of a number of DLC coatings against UHMWPE in water

Fig. 8.4 Comparative friction characteristics of different materials for hip joint couples

It was not possible to measure wear of the UHMWPE during these tests, but tests run in parallel at other laboratories found no significant reduction in UHMWPE wear by using the coating **(4)**. Without the reduction of friction or wear, the efficiency of DLC coatings in metal-on-UHMWPE bearings was in doubt.

The low friction and wear of the Graphit-iC coating against hard counterparts was likely to be of more use in a metal-on-metal hip joint. A series of tests performed at Teer Coatings Limited, using Graphit-iC coated CoCrMo pins and flats sliding in water at 3 mm s^{-1}, gave very promising results. A load of 40 N on a 5 mm diameter hemispherically ended pin was chosen to exert the highest possible contact pressure without causing severe plastic deformation of the CoCrMo substrate material. This provided a mean Hertzian contact pressure of 1.4 GPa and did cause a little plastic deformation as can be seen in Fig. 8.5(a). The wear scar on the coated pin [Fig. 8.5(b)] was measured every 10 000 cycles which allowed the progressive wear of the coated pin to be measured.

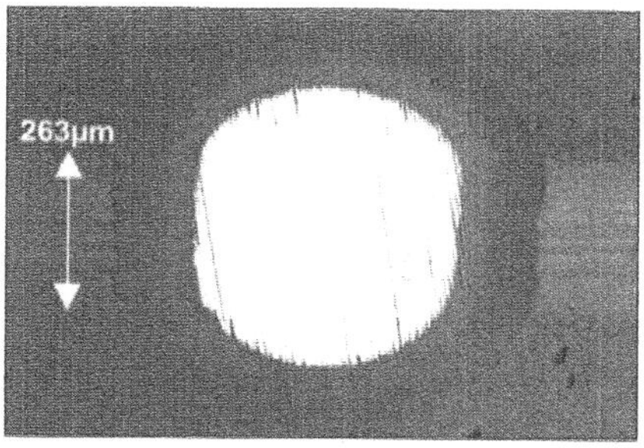

(a) Ball crater on the flat wear track after 50 000 cycles

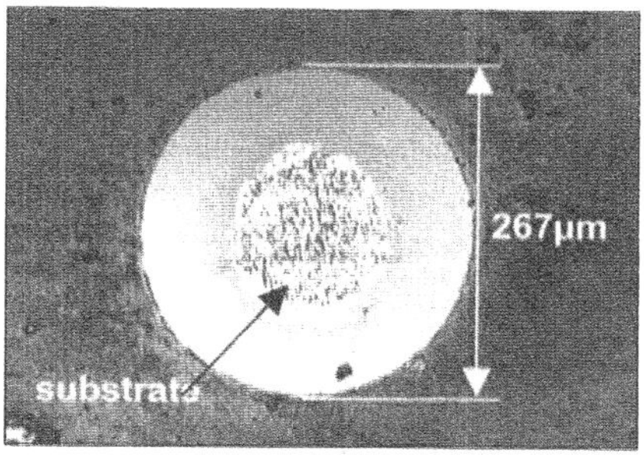

(b) Wear scar on the coated pin after 50 000 cycles

Fig. 8.5

After 40 000 cycles the coating on the pin had worn through to the Cr interlayer, and the CoCrMo was exposed after 50 000 cycles as can be seen above. The friction coefficient during the tests was stable at ~0.03 and the steady-state wear rate of the coated pin was 5 ×

10^{-18} m^3 N^{-1} m^{-1}. The wear of the coated flat was not measurable but there is nothing to suggest that it would be any worse than that of the pin, so a combined wear rate of 1×10^{-17} m^3 N^{-1} m^{-1} could be assumed.

Tests using uncoated CoCrMo pins and flats at a reduced load of 5 N (mean Hertzian contact pressure of 0.7 GPa) in water produced a friction coefficient of 0.4, but the load was high enough to deform the CoCrMo and make wear quantification by geometric measurement very difficult. Streicher *et al.* **(10)** reported that the best wear and friction results were found with high carbon content (0.2–0.3 wt.% C) fine grain structured (wrought as opposed to cast) CoCrMo alloys running in serum and providing average friction coefficients of ~0.2 ($0.1 < \mu < 0.45$) and specific wear rates of $\sim 2 \times 10^{-15}$ m^3 N^{-1} m^{-1}. They used Hertzian contact pressures of ~1 GPa and 10 mm s^{-1} sliding speed – perhaps explaining the lower coefficients of friction, but they also reported that the lower carbon content (0.05–0.08 wt.% C) material did not show significant differences in friction, and found very little difference in friction and wear when using serum or water.

This suggests an improvement in wear of 400 times and a reduction in friction by 75 per cent when comparing the Graphit-iC to the CoCrMo directly. If the CoCrMo heads and cups wear from 2–20 μm per year **(8)** the Graphit-iC coated heads and cups could wear as little as 0.05 μm per year and give potential lifetimes of up to 50 years. This would provide a considerable reduction in wear debris which would be mainly carbon and therefore inherently safe within the human body. A reduction in friction by 75 per cent should also significantly reduce the stress at the implant-bone interface and thereby, the possibility of implant loosening.

Friction measurement tests performed at the University of Leeds, to determine the performance of Graphit-iC in serum, recorded a friction coefficient of 0.25, at a contact pressure of 2.83 MPa. (A load of 20 N was applied to Graphit-iC coated pins with a 3 mm diameter flat that provided conformal contact.) Friction was higher than that found for coated hemispherical pins in water ($\mu \sim 0.03$, 1.41 GPa mean Hertzian contact) and was thought to be due to the serum and the conformal contact. Tests in serum, performed at TCL with coated hemispherical 5 mm diameter pins (non-conformal contact) at loads of 40 N and 4 N produced friction coefficients of 0.07 and 0.12 at mean Hertzian contact pressures of 1.41 GPa and 0.65 GPa respectively. This demonstrates a variation of friction with contact pressure, as has been shown for solid lubricants **(15)**, and also a difference between water and serum. It was, therefore, concluded that it would be necessary to measure the friction of the heads and cups in serum to determine the exact level of friction.

The reciprocating wear tests conducted on pins and plates at Leeds produced coating failure. Of the three pairs of pins and flats, two failed completely after 24 hours, but the other survived with no measurable wear. The wear tracks produced were ball cratered at the ends to assess the type of failure.

The ball crater on the failed coating [Fig. 8.6(a)] showed a brittle type of fracture at the edge of the worn area. The failure appeared to have occurred at either the coating interface with the substrate, or within the substrate, just below this interface. This was not failure by progressive wear, as no preliminary evidence of failure is evident in Fig. 8.6(b). Figure 8.6(b) shows the same position on the wear track of the coating that survived the test. In this case no wear of the coating can be measured. The reason of failure was thought to be due to the lack of conformal contact due to the misalignment of the pin and flat.

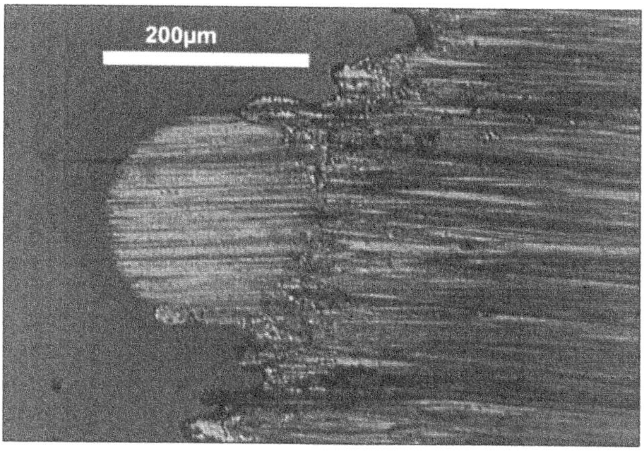

(a) A coating that failed

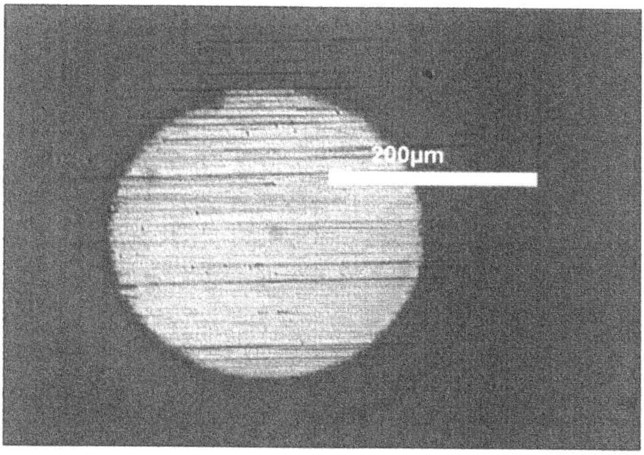

(b) The coating that survived the four 24 h periods

Fig. 8.6 Ball craters at the ends of reciprocating wear tracks

Tests were performed on a series of heads and cups coated with Graphit-iC. The pairs had been manufactured to have varied radial clearances (50, 100, 150, 300, and 550 μm), to provide different contact geometries. A larger 53 mm diameter pairing with 50 μm radial clearance was also included. Figure 8.7 shows the results when the two extreme clearances of the 28 mm diameter pairs, and a 53 mm diameter pair were used to record friction in the Leeds driven pendulum test, and also compared to other material pairings.

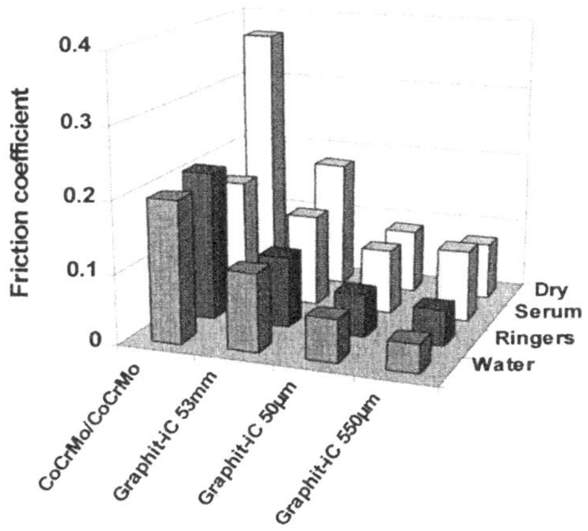

(a) Graphit-iC coated and a commercial uncoated CoCrMo hip in different lubricants

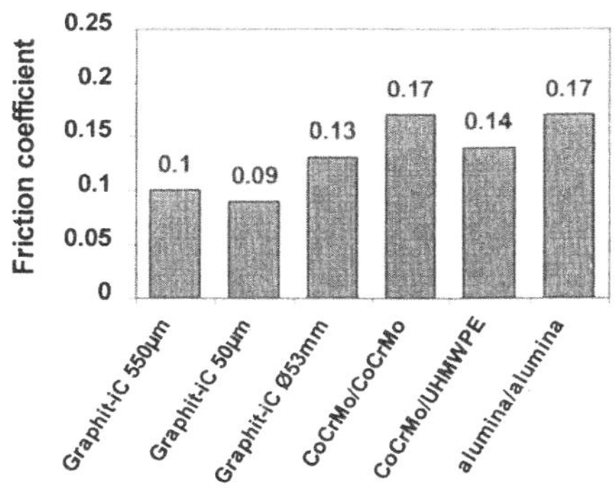

(b) Graphit-iC with different radial clearances and other material pairings in serum

Fig. 8.7 Friction values in the driven pendulum test rig

It can be seen in Fig. 8.7(a) that the Graphit-iC coated pairs produced lower friction values in all fluids. It also shows that the 550 μm clearance (highest contact pressure) gave the lowest friction in all fluids except the serum. The serum appears to contradict the trend showing lowest friction in the 28 mm diameter 50 μm clearance pair. It also benefits the CoCrMo pair, providing more lubrication than the other fluids. The difference in friction between these tests and the pin-on-flat tests suggest that the contact pressure and geometry should be matched to that found in heads and cups, to enable different material pairings to be compared in simple bench tests.

When tested in the physiological simulator the coating performance was not as expected. The tests were stopped prematurely as there was evidence of failure in all but one pair, indicated by the serum turning dark in colour due to small particles of coating. These failures occurred after differing numbers of cycles. There was no way of determining the exact moment of failure during the test, as the tests were checked after approximately every 100 000 cycles. The duration up to the last check was the only estimate that could be made of the coating durability, and these values are shown in Table 8.1.

Table 8.1 Lifetimes of Graphit-iC coated heads and cups in simulator tests

Radial clearance (μm)	*Period before failure (× 100 000 cycles)*	*Final condition of coating*
50	0	Coating removed
100	4	Coating removed
150	>1.92 (no failure)	Intact
300	1	Coating removed
550	5	Coating removed

The heads and cups with 150 μm and 300 μm clearance were run together and both stopped after 192 000 cycles as the 300 μm clearance pair appeared to have failed. When they were examined after the tests it was again observed that the coating had failed in a similar way to the pin-on-plate tests. The failed head was ball cratered at the edge of the worn area and the fractured coating can be seen in Fig. 8.8(a). The 150 μm clearance head showed no signs of wear, without even the slightest scratch. This head was ball cratered, Fig. 8.8(b), which allowed the coating thickness to be measured: no reduction in thickness was found.

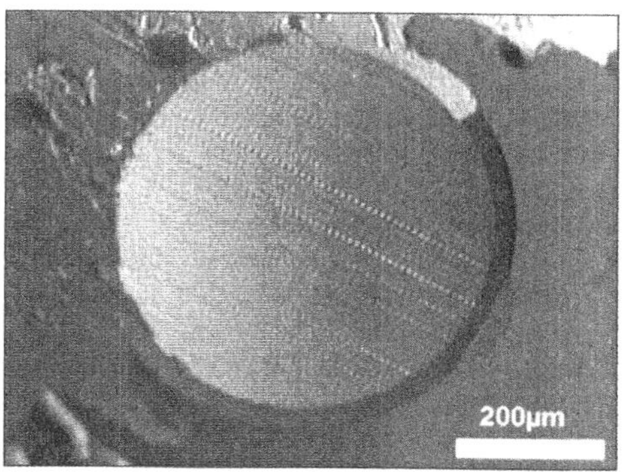

(a) The failed coating of the 300 μm clearance head

Fig. 8.8 Ball craters, both after 192 000 cycles

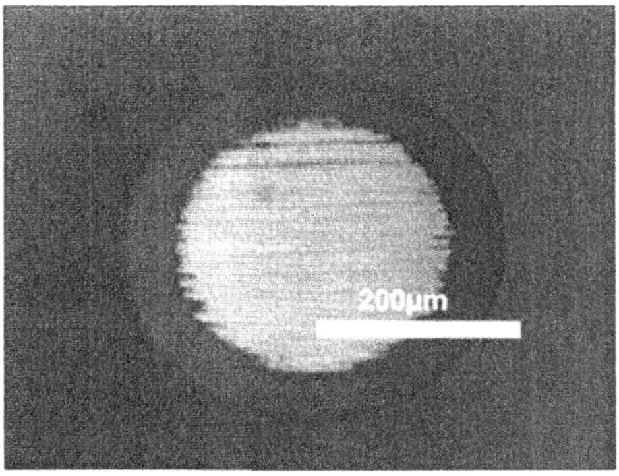

(b) The intact coating of the 150 µm clearance head

Fig. 8.8 Ball craters, both after 192 000 cycles (cont.)

The mode of failure appeared to be an adhesion type of coating failure rather than the progressive wear that would be expected. However, the adhesion of the coatings was not found to be inferior as determined by a standard scratch test performed on an area of coating next to the failed area on the 300 µm clearance head.

This suggested a type of failure not previously observed for the Graphit-iC coating. The mean Hertzian contact pressures for the heads and cups did not appear to be excessive for the coating. The standard pin-on-disc tests, at TCL, using coated M42 steel and WC balls produce Hertzian contact pressures in excess of 3 GPa, whereas the coated CoCrMo heads and cups produce a maximum contact pressure of 230 MPa on the 550 µm clearance pair, and 47 MPa for the 50 µm clearance pair [calculated using the ball-on-plane model with an equivalent radius (**16**)]. If there was misalignment of the head and cup it may have been possible for the contact stress to exceed these values, and those permitted by the coating, resulting in the type of failure shown. The coating on CoCrMo would not be as compliant as UHMWPE or uncoated CoCrMo, where some misalignment could be tolerated via bulk deformation.

Another possible cause of failure could have been due to the repetitive cyclic loading produced in the simulator, resulting in a type of fatigue failure near to the coating/substrate interface. However, the cyclic nature of the load was not thought to be dissimilar to that found during a high load pin-on-disc test, where the coating and substrate experience elastic deformation as the pin moves around the wear track. The short duration of some of the tests was not thought to be long enough for fatigue failures to occur.

These results highlight the differences between accelerated bench tests and simulator testing. Further development of the Graphit-iC coating will require longer duration wear testing with geometries closer to those found in hip joints, to try to induce the type of failure shown here. The simulator testing procedure does not allow the performance of the coated bearing to be monitored and makes detailed analysis after the failure more difficult. It is difficult to measure wear following catastrophic coating failure. Once the mode of failure is understood steps can be taken to improve the performance of the coatings in the metal-on-metal hip prostheses application.

It was also impossible to draw any conclusions on the effect of radial clearance in the heads and cups tested as the nature of the coating failure was not considered to be dependant on this parameter.

8.4 Conclusions

Simple laboratory pin-on-flat wear tests indicated a higher coefficient of friction for the carbon coating Graphit-iC sliding against UHMWPE in water than for uncoated CoCrMo.

Pin-on-flat tests have shown that Graphit-iC/Graphit-iC bearing contacts can produce friction coefficients of 0.03 and a wear rate of 5×10^{-18} m^3 N^{-1} m^{-1} when tested in water compared to a coefficient of 0.2–0.4 and a wear rate of 2×10^{-15} m^3 N^{-1} m^{-1} for CoCrMo/CoCrMo **(10)**. When tested in serum the friction coefficient was increased to 0.07.

Graphit-iC coated CoCrMo heads and cups produced lower coefficients of friction than metal-on-metal, metal/UHMWPE and ceramic/ceramic material pairings when tested in serum.

Physiological simulator tests produced catastrophic coating failure in some hip joint pairs, but one pair survived and showed no signs of wear whatsoever.

The wear resistance and low friction still provide excellent potential for the carbon coatings in the application of hip prostheses, but new simple configuration test methods are required to further improve the coating performance before full term simulator tests can be utilized to the full.

Acknowledgements

The authors would like to thank the DTI, DoH, and EPSRC for support as part of LINK Surface Engineering Projects; Prof. Santu Datta and Redha Touaitia at the University of Northumbria for structural analysis of coatings; Prof. John Fisher, Paul Firkins, Devon Derby, and Hanna Marrs of the University of Leeds for testing; John Egan and 3M Healthcare for materials supply and wear testing; and Avatar Medical Limited for providing the metal-on-metal hips.

References

(1) **Wang, A., Stark, C.,** and **Dumbleton, J. H.** Mechanistic and morphological origins of ultra high molecular weight polyethylene wear debris in total joint replacement prostheses. In Advances in Medical Tribology, MEP Limited, 1998, 1–15.

(2) **Willert, H. G.** and **Buchhorn, G. H.** Particle disease due to wear of UHMWPE. Biological, material and mechanical considerations of joint replacement (Ed. B. F. Morrey), 1993, 87–102 (Raven Press, New York).

(3) **Monaghan, D. P., Teer, D. G., Logan, P. A., Efeoglu, I.,** and **Arnell, R. D.** Deposition of wear resistant coatings based on DLC by unbalanced magnetron sputtering. Surf. Coat. Tech., 60 (1993), 525–530.

(4) **Pickard, J., Fisher, J., Gibbons, D., Koybayashi, H., Ito, A., Tateishi, T., Jones, A., Teer, D.,** and **Egan, J.** Multi-centred tribological testing of UHMWPE against DLC coatings on cobalt chromium alloys. Presented at the World Biomaterials Congress, Hawaii 2000, to be published in J. Biomed. Mater. Res.

(5) **Jones, A. H. S., Camino, D., Jiang, J.,** and **Teer, D. G.** Novel high wear resistant coatings deposited by magnetron sputtering of carbon targets. J. Eng. Tribol. 1998, 212, 301–306.

(6) **Camino, D., Jones, A. H. S., Mercs, D.,** and **Teer, D. G.** High performance sputtered carbon coatings for wear resistant applications. Vacuum, 52, (1999) 125–131.

(7) **Lappalainen, R., Anttila, A.,** and **Heinonen, H.** Diamond coated total hip replacements. Clinical Orthopaedics and Related Research. No. 352. Lippincott-Raven publishers 1998, 118–127.

(8) **Semlitsch, M.** and **Willert, H. G.** Clinical wear behaviour of UHMWPE cups paired with metal and ceramic ball heads in comparison to metal-on-metal pairings of hip joint replacements. In Advances in Medical Tribology, MEP Limited, 1998, 165–180.

(9) **Rieker, C. B., Kottig, P., Schon, R., Windler, M.,** and **Wyss, U. P.** Clinical wear performance of metal-on-metal hip arthroplasties. In alternative bearing surfaces in total joint replacement, ASTM, STP 1346, J. J. Jacobs and T. L. Craig, ASTM, 1998.

(10) **Streicher, R. M., Semlitsch, M., Schon, R., Weber, H.,** and **Rieker, C.** Metal-on-metal articulation for artificial hip joints: laboratory study and clinical results. In Advances in Medical Tribology, MEP Limited, 1998, 83–92.

(11) **Jiang, J., Arnell, R. D.,** and **Tong, J.** Some special tribological features of DLC coatings on soft substrates. Wear, 211 (1997), 254–264.

(12) **Bellido-González, V., Hampshire, J., Jones, A. H. S., Witts, J., Allen, T. J., Teer, D. G.,** and **Pierret, B.** Advances in the analysis and characterisation of DLC coatings. Surface and Coatings Technology 98 (1998), 1272–1279.

(13) **von Stebut, J., Michel, H., Bellido-González, V.,** and **Jones, A. H. S.** Ball cratering: a versatile tool for first order surface coating characterisation. Paper presented at the PSE Conference, Garmisch Partenkirchen, Germany, 1996.

(14) **Dowson, D.** and **Jobbins, B.** Design and development of a versatile hip joint simulator. J. Engng In Medicine, 1988, 17, 1–6.

(15) **Bowden, F. P.** and **Tabor, D.** The Friction and Lubrication of Solids, Part 2, (Clarendon Press, Oxford, 1964), P214.

(16) **Jin, Z. M., Dowson, D.,** and **Fisher, J.** Analysis of fluid film lubrication in artificial hip joint replacements with surfaces of high elastic modulus. Proc. IMechE 1997, Vol. 211, Part H, 247–256.

A H S Jones, S K Taylor, D G Teer, and **M Elloy**
Teer Coatings Limited, Hartlebury, UK

9

Simulator Testing of Total Knee Replacements

G W Blunn, C J Bell, P S Walker, S Chatterjee, J Perry, P Campbell, H Haider, and J P Paul

Abstract

In order to determine the effect of improvements in design and materials on wear of total knee replacement, a valid test method is required. This test method should reproduce the wear patterns seen on retrieved knee replacements. We have tested various designs of implants using a force-control knee simulator and analysed the wear on these implants. The tests were conducted in 50 per cent bovine serum for up to ten million cycles. On condylar replacements, wear was associated with scratching and burnishing. Wear rates between different designs could be discriminated. Delamination wear occurred only in those samples which had been artificially aged. Tests showed that wear on a meniscal knee design equalled that, or was greater than that, observed on a condylar design. On meniscal designs wear was associated mainly with the meniscal bearing surface.

9.1 Introduction

Recent advances in knee replacement design and polyethylene processing can potentially extend durability of total knee replacements (TKR) **(1)**. However, in order to verify the effect of these perceived improvements a realistic and valid test method is required. Specifications of the method are that it should be reproducible by different laboratories, and that results should be obtainable within six months and be applicable to various designs of total knee replacement. These designs include fixed-axis, rotating hinges, fixed-bearing condylar designs of varying constraint, and rotating platform or mobile bearings. It is important that wear patterns produced in the simulator resemble those on retrieved implants. We have proposed a test scheme where representative walking forces and moments are input, as well as flexion–extension, the other motions being determined by the laxity of the implant, but with simulated soft tissue restraint built-in to obtain realistic displacements and rotations. This test scheme is accomplished using a Stanmore knee wear test simulator **(2)**. This Chapter describes the results of long-term testing using this method.

9.2 Description of the knee simulator

In the four-station knee simulator a walking cycle is imposed on the joint by applying the flexion and extension angle, the axial compressive force, the anterior–posterior (AP) shear force, and the internal and external torques. The input values were adapted from the work of Morrison **(3)**, and Taylor *et al.* **(4)**. The replicate, realistic variations in the axial force, with a ten per cent random variation, were applied. The force and motion data are specified in the draft standard ISO/CD 14243-1 **(5)**. The femoral component was mounted in a fixture such that its flexion and extension axis was along the average centre of curvature of the arc extending from the distal to the posterior femoral condyle. The femur was constrained to move only around this axis. The tibial component was free to move in a horizontal plane and to rotate about a vertical axis.

The AP force and the torque were applied by pneumatic cylinders. To provide a similar restraint between the femoral and tibial components, as would occur in the natural knee, springs connecting the frame of the machine to the tibial dish were used to simulate the passive soft tissues. These springs provided resistance to AP and rotational movements. In the knee where a cruciate ligament was preserved, full strength springs were used. For cruciate ligament resection, the spring stiffness was reduced to one-third. The data for the stiffness were obtained from Fukubayashi *et al.* **(6)**. A photograph of the knee simulator which is made by Instron Corp. is shown in Fig. 9.1. The schematic of the design is shown in Fig. 9.2. The physiologic input cycles are shown in Fig. 9.3. During a test, the forces and displacements were monitored using a computer.

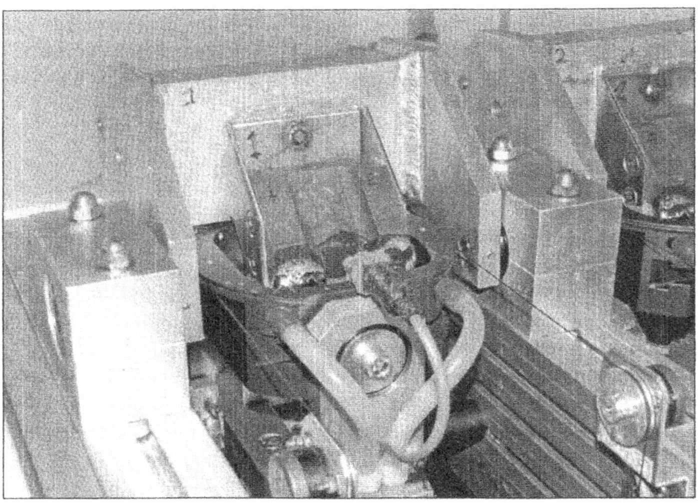

Fig. 9.1 Photograph of the Stanmore knee simulator – single station

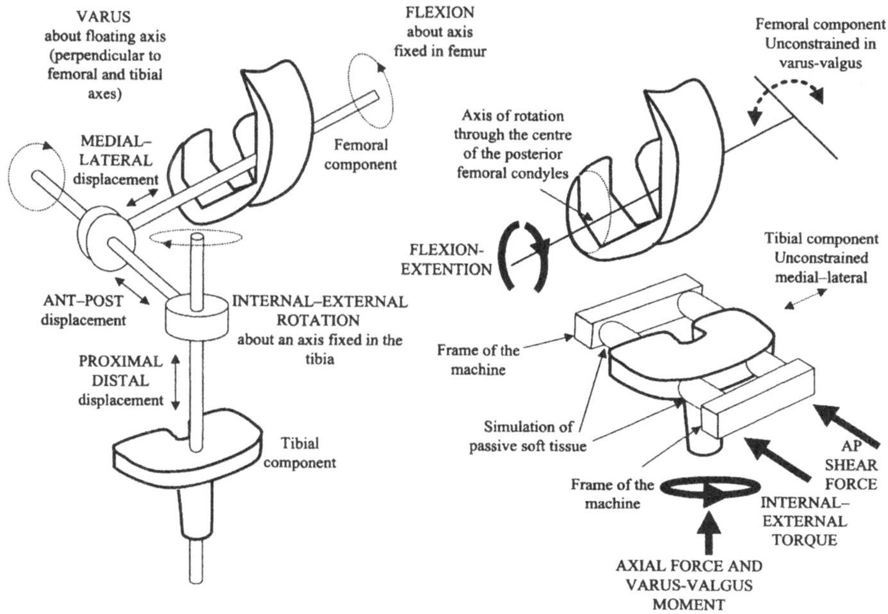

Fig. 9.2 Schematic of the Stanmore knee simulator

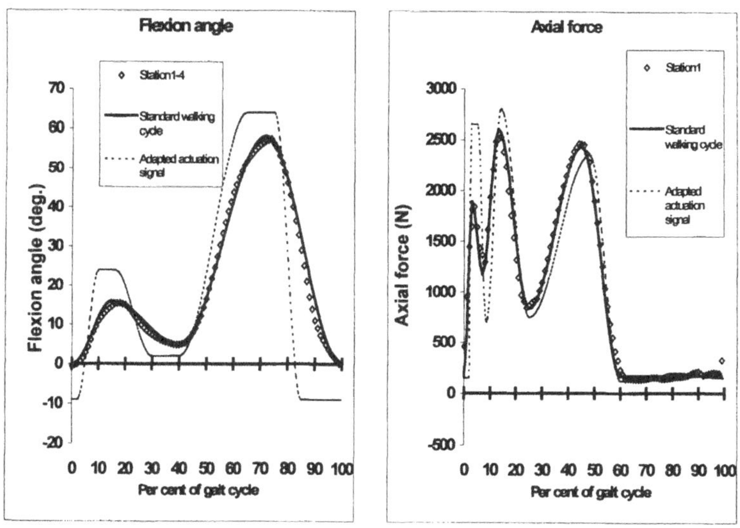

Fig. 9.3 Input loads and motions for standard walking cycle and enhanced duty cycle – the graphs also show the response to the actuator motions and inputs of individual stations

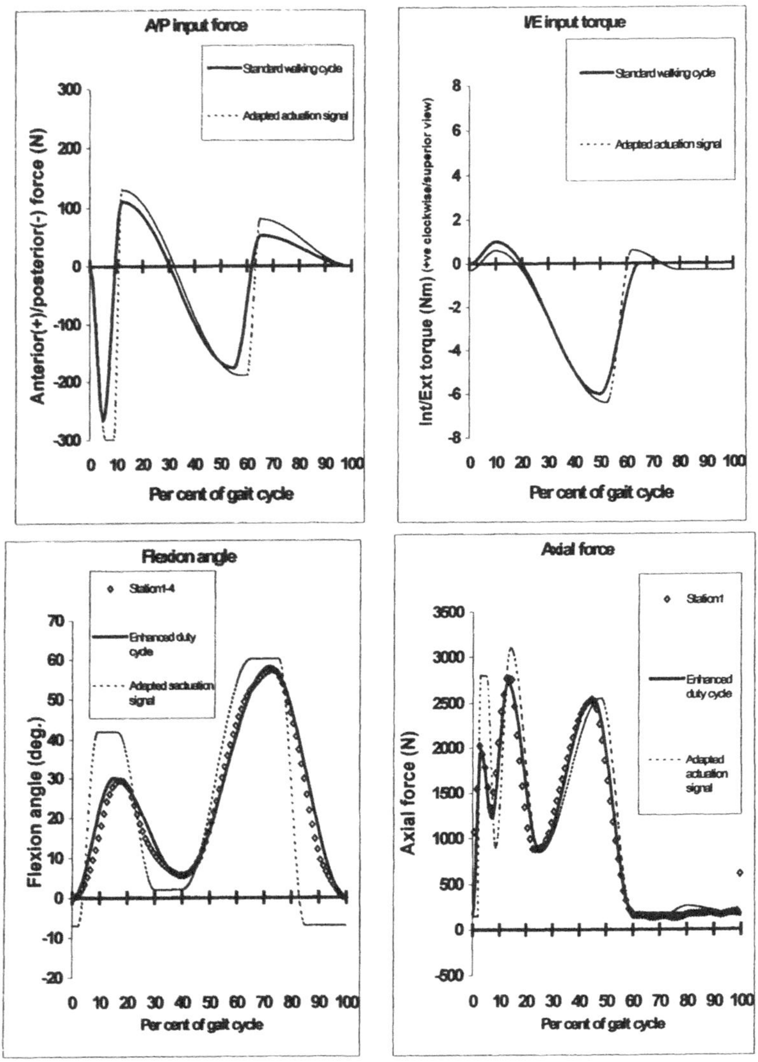

Fig. 9.3 Input loads and motions for standard walking cycle and enhanced duty cycle – the graphs also show the response to the actuator motions and inputs of individual stations (cont.)

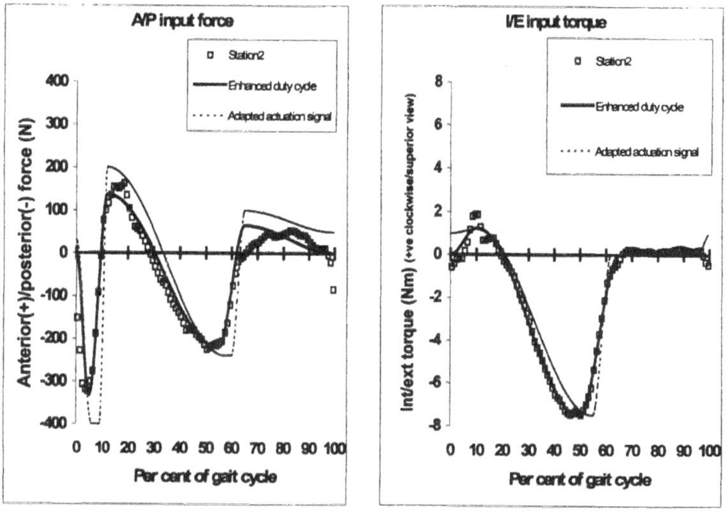

Fig. 9.3 Input loads and motions for standard walking cycle and enhanced duty cycle – the graphs also show the response to the actuator motions and inputs of individual stations (cont.)

9.3 Test methodology

In the first test two kinematic and two IB2 knees were used, sterilized by gamma irradiation in air. The test was run at 1 Hz with 50 per cent calf serum at 37 °C, and wear depth measurements and fluid samples were taken every one million cycles. The fluid samples were processed to isolate polyethylene debris particles and the shape and size distributions of the particles were analysed **(7)**. One sample of each knee was artificially aged in an oxygen chamber for 0.25 days after two, three, four, and five million cycles. At nine million cycles, the components were aged for four days. At 10.7 million cycles, the un-oxidized components were replaced with two kinemax components aged in oxygen for six days. The test was ended after a total of 11.3 million cycles. An SEM was used to study the surfaces.

In the second test two force-actuated four station knee simulators were used for testing. Two designs of knee were used. These were the NexGen and the MBK designs. Two knees of each design were subjected to the standard walking cycle which is the current ISO standard for knee simulator testing. Two other knees of each design were subjected to an enhanced duty cycle aimed to reproduce more extreme loading conditions experienced during everyday activities. This was achieved by increasing axial force associated with an increase in flexion angle. The enhanced duty cycle may be representative of walking up a slope. A comparison of the standard walking cycle with the enhanced duty cycle is shown in Fig. 9.3. This test ran for a total of five million cycles. At intervals of one million cycles, the weight loss of the tibial polymer component was measured and the displacements and rotations of the tibial component were determined. At the end of the test the articulating surfaces were inspected for wear.

9.4 Results

In the first test the polymer components developed wear patches which steadily increased in depth with time. Wear scars on the polymer showed burnishing and multiple fine scratching (Fig. 9.4), while the femoral components showed scratching. The depth of the wear track for the kinematic knee was about three times that of the IB2 (Fig. 9.5). There was no delamination wear or subsurface cracking up to nine million cycles. Particles isolated from the serum were characterized as flakes, granules, or fibrils (Fig. 9.6). Particle analysis showed more granules and fewer fibrils for the kinematic knee, with smaller particle dimensions. After 10.7 million cycles, one kinematic joint showed surface blistering and subsurface cracking within a heavily oxidized band (Fig. 9.7). At 11.3 million cycles (i.e. 0.6 million running with the kinemax), one kinemax knee showed delamination to approximately 1 mm depth, the extent of heavy oxidation (Fig. 9.8). A section through the component, stained with chlorosulphonic acid to indicate regions of oxidation, showed high oxidation near the surface, as observed in retrievals.

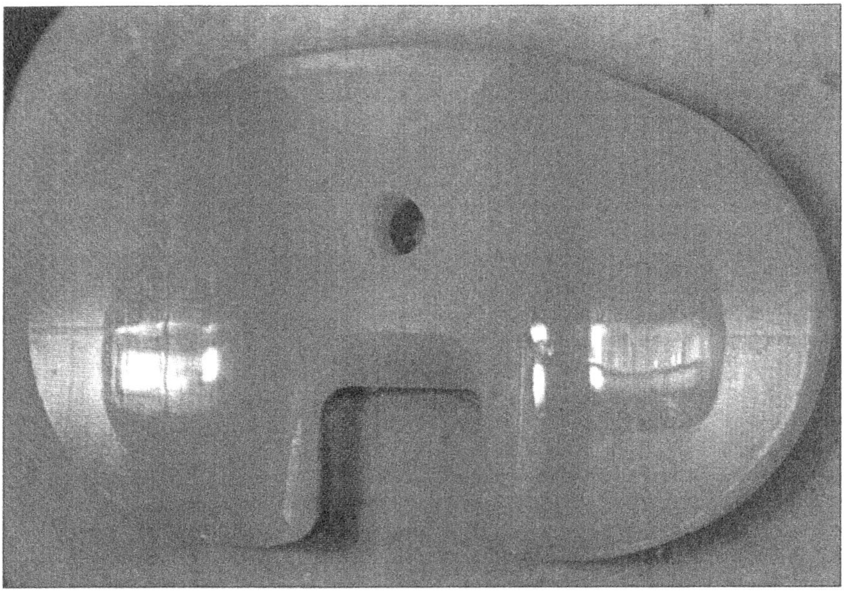

Fig. 9.4 Photograph of kinematic component at five million cycles

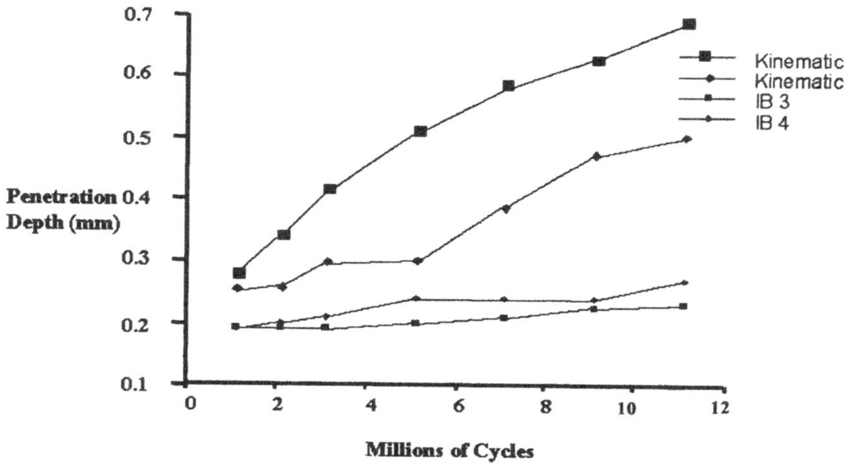

Fig. 9.5 Penetration depth (medial condyle)

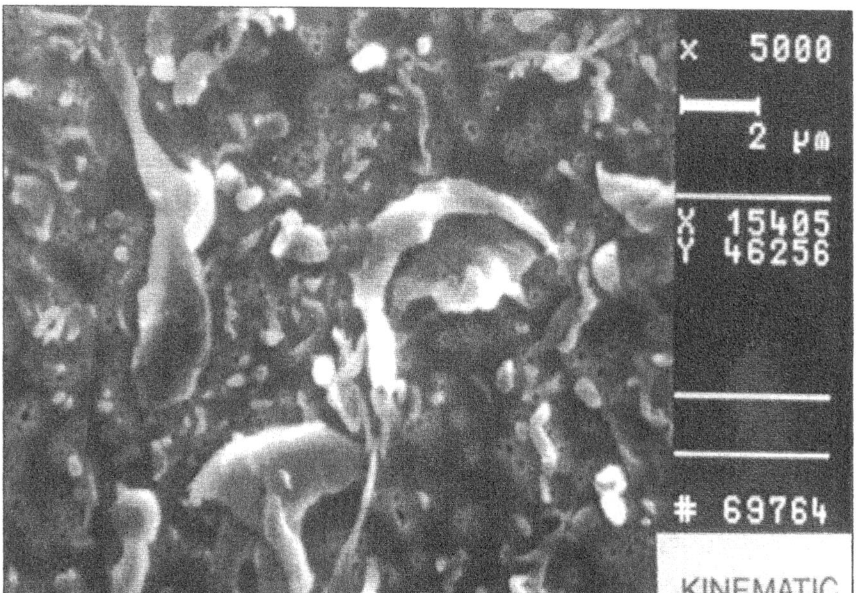

Fig. 9.6 SEM of isolated particles taken from the serum of kinematic knee replacement at five million cycles – note the granules (G), flakes (F), and fibrils (Fi)

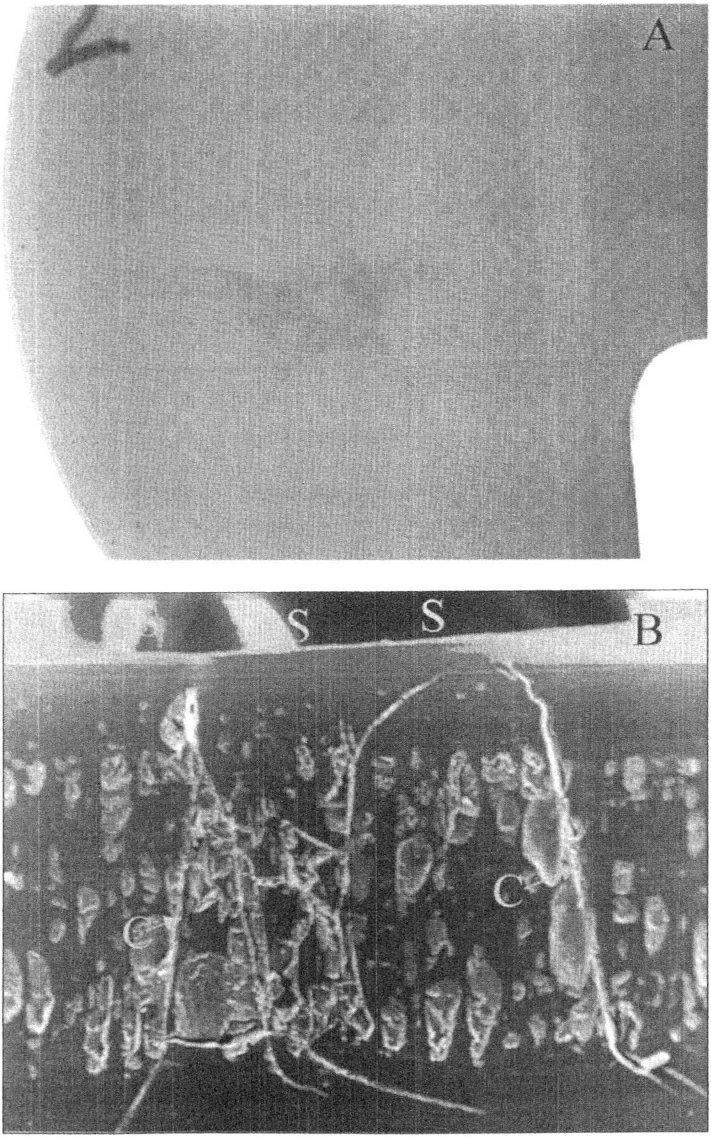

Fig. 9.7 Photograph of kinematic component showing cracking of the UHMWPE after 10 million cycles – (A) SEM of a section through this component (in B) showing surface of the wear track (S) and multiple cracks (C)

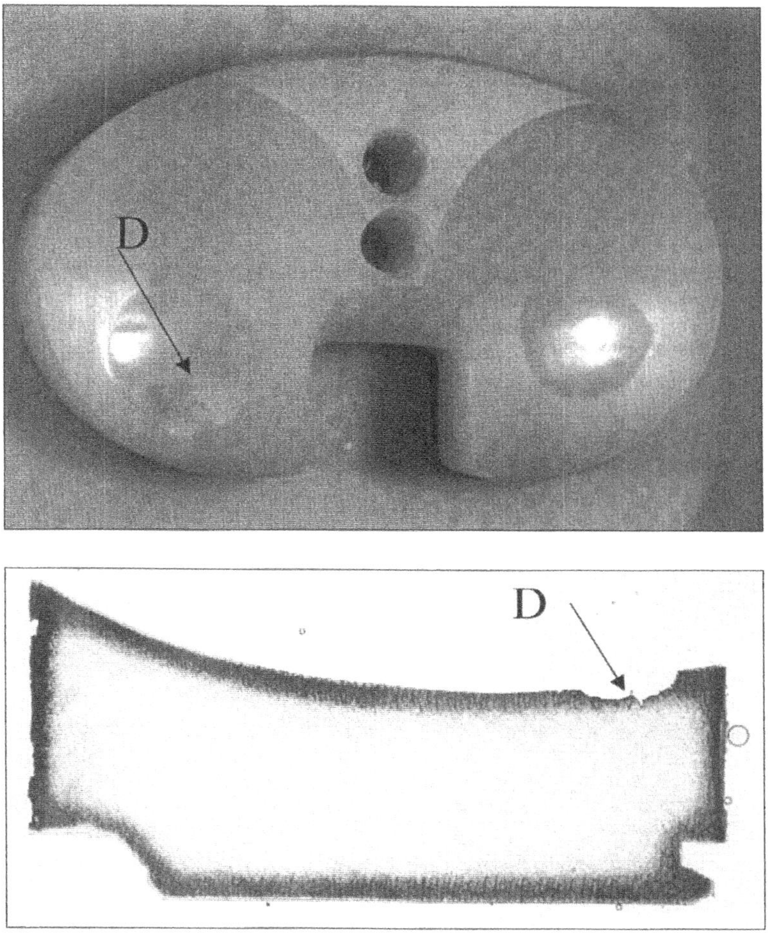

Fig. 9.8 Photograph of kinemax showing delamination (D) and a section through the component which has been stained with chlorosulphonic acid, turning the oxidized plastic brown

The NexGen and MBK designs were used in the second test. The MBK tibial plate is free to move on its meniscal surface and dislocation is prevented by metallic stops. The kinematic knee showed greater initial motion for the mobile bearing designs. However, this motion decreased with time and became erratic. The MBK demonstrated a slip–stick motion which varied between cycles. Figure 9.9 shows internal/external rotation for the implants during the enhanced duty cycle at four and five million cycles. One of the MBKs moved more freely at five million than at four million cycles. In both tests the motions of the NexGen were consistent with time, showing an increase in motion as the test progressed, due to decreased conformity caused by creep and wear of the polyethylene insert. Tibial components subjected to the standard walking cycle lost similar amounts of weight. After five million cycles there was no significant difference between the two, with both designs losing 24 mg every one million cycles. Wear of the NexGen TKR was similar under the two wear regimes. However, overall wear of the MBK TKR was greater for the enhanced duty cycle regime (Fig. 9.10). Initially there was no difference in the wear of the MBK polymer compared to the NexGen in the enhanced duty cycle. However, after two million cycles the wear rate of the MBK increased and at five million cycles there was a 50 per cent difference. Due to rolling of the femoral component, the wear tracks on the tibial surface of the NexGen (Fig. 9.9) were longer than the measured AP movement with tracks measuring around 23 mm in anterior to posterior length for both the walking cycle and the enhanced duty cycle. The wear tracks on the tibial surface of the NexGen TKRs were more discernible than the wear tracks on the MBK TKRs. Although wear was evident on the surface of the MBK TKR as a burnished wear track, most of the wear occurred on the meniscal surface. On the meniscal surface wear occurred in large patches and was evident as burnished areas together with radial scratches. Scanning electron microscopy of the under-surface showed scratches in the polyethylene and adhesive wear characterized by ripples in the polymer (Fig. 9.11). There was no evidence of the original machining marks on this surface. The corresponding surface on the alloy tibial base plate for the MBK was heavily scratched (Fig. 9.11). These scratches were radial. There were also regions where patchy transfer films of polyethylene occurred. All of these features could be identified on the MBK at five million cycles from both the enhanced duty cycle and the standard walking cycle.

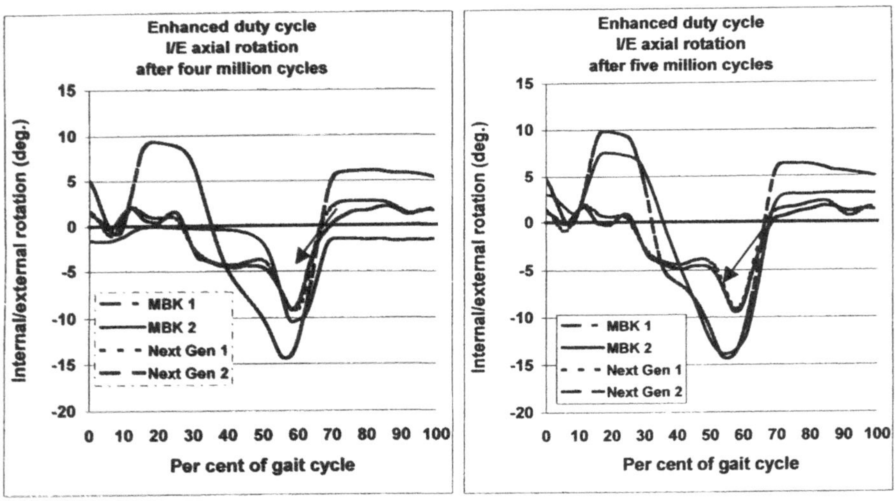

Fig. 9.9 Internal–external rotations at four million cycles and five million cycles for the enhanced duty cycle – note how one of the MBKs moves less freely than the other at four million cycles, but after five million cycles movement is similar (arrowed)

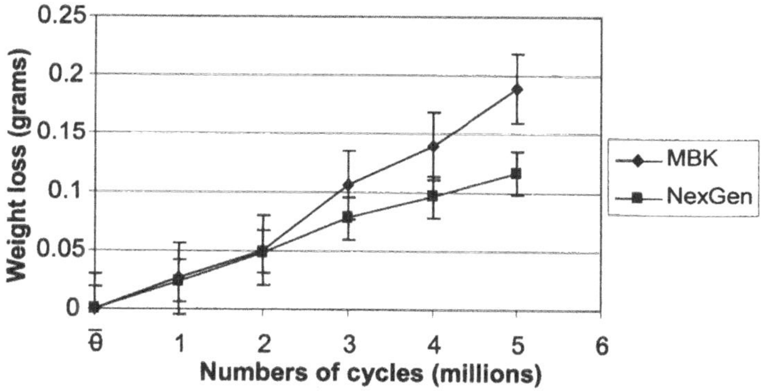

Fig. 9.10 Weight loss of the MBK and NexGen after five million cycles

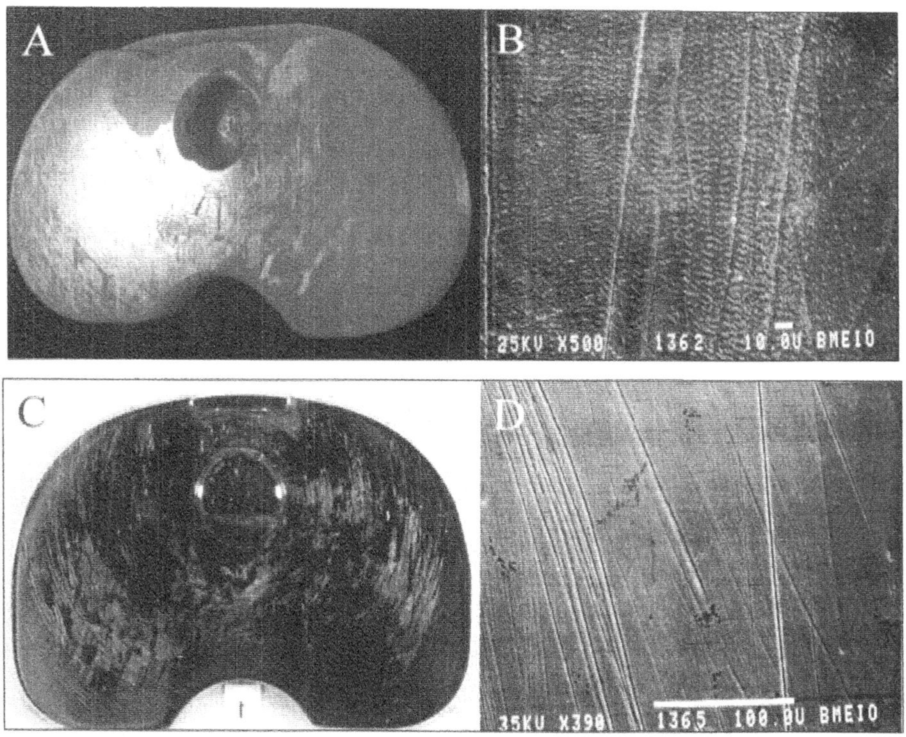

Fig. 9.11 Meniscal bearing surface of MBK after five million enhanced duty cycles showing adhesive wear and scratching (A and B) – surface of MBK base plate showing radial scratches and transfer film evident as refractive regions on the alloy surface (B and C)

9.5 Discussion and conclusions

The first test reported in this Chapter demonstrates that the locations and extent of the wear areas were consistent with those observed in retrievals, but neither pitting nor delamination were observed in the nine million cycle test, despite artificial ageing. However this ageing produced far less oxidation and at greater depth than that seen in ten year retrievals. On the other hand, artificial ageing of one component produced delamination at 10.7 million cycles. However, when the ageing produced oxidation at a depth of approximately 1 mm below the surface, delamination occurred after 0.6 million cycles. Theory indicated that delamination was due to sub-surface crack propagation from accumulated shear damage. Hence the lack of pitting and delamination in the nine million cycle test was due to inadequate test duration, or more likely to the absence of sufficient oxidation, which degrades the mechanical properties to make fatigue damage more likely. Debris particle sizes were consistent with those reported in retrieved tissue, but with fewer larger particles **(7)**. The latter are likely to be associated with pitting and delamination. It was concluded that artificial ageing may be needed to reproduce long-term *in vivo* behavior and will also exaggerate the difference between polyethylenes with different resistances to oxidative degradation **(8)**.

The second test reported in this Chapter demonstrates the effect of design on the wear of the tibial polymer component. The stick-slip motion associated with the MBK occurs during prolonged testing. This is associated with changing lubrication conditions during the test. This results in increased wear at the lower bearing surface, scratching of the tibial base plate and the production of transfer films. The MBK showed a significant increase in wear (at one million cycles) for the enhanced compared to standard walking cycle. However, there was a smaller increase in the wear rate for the condylar components. This study proposes that particular designs of TKR may wear and behave differently depending on the input cycles. Standard walking cycles are needed to represent normal activity. However, this does not produce more catastrophic wear mechanisms within a feasible period of testing. An enhanced cycle should highlight weaknesses in the design in a shorter time.

Acknowledgements

This work was funded by Medical Devices Agency, Department of Health, UK, and a consortium of manufacturers. Orthopaedic Hospital, Los Angeles, USA. University of Strathclyde, Glasgow, UK.

References

(1) **Blunn, G. W., Brach del Preva, E., Costa, L., Fisher, J.,** and **Freeman, M. A. R.** The fabrication, sterilization and wear of UHMWPE for total knee replacement. *J. Bone Joint Surg* (2002) (in press).

(2) **Walker, P. S., Blunn, G. W., Broom, D. R., Perry, J., Watkins, A., Sathasivam, S., Dewar, M. E.,** and **Paul, J. P.** A knee simulating machine for performance evaluation of total knee replacements. *J. Biomechanics*, 1997, **30**, 83–89.

(3) **Morrison, J. B.** The mechanics of the knee joint in relation to normal walking. *J. Biomechanics*, 1970, **3**, 51–61.

(4) **Taylor, S. J. G., Walker, P. S., Perry, J., Cannon, S. R.,** and **Woledge, R.** The forces in the distal femur and the knee during walking and other activities measured by telemetry. *J. Arthroplasty,* 1998, **13**, 428–437.
(5) ISO/CD 14243-1. Implants for surgery, wear of total knee joint prosthesis, Part 1 – loading and displacement parameters for wear testing machines with low control and corresponding environmental conditions for tests. *London, International Organisation for Standardisation,* 1998.
(6) **Fukubayashi, T., Torzilli, P. A., Sherman, M. F.,** and **Warren, R. F.** An *in vitro* biomechanical evaluation of anterior-posterior motion of the knee. Tibial displacement, rotation and torque. *J. Bone Joint Surg.*, 1982, **64A**, 258–264.
(7) **Beaule, P. E., Campbell, P. A., Walker, P. S., Schmalzried, T. P., Dorey, F. J., Blunn, G. W., Bell, C. J., Yahia, L'H.,** and **Amstutz, H. C.** Polyethylene wear characteristics *in vivo* and in a knee simulator. *J. Biomed. Mater.* Res., 2002, **60**, 411–419.
(8) **Walker, P. S., Blunn, G. W., Perry, J. P., Bell, C. J., Sathasivam, S., Andriacchi, T. P., Paul, J. P., Haider, H.,** and **Campbell, P. A.** Methodology for long-term wear testing of total knee replacements. *Clin. Orthop.*, 1999, **372**, 290–301.

G W Blunn, C J Bell, P S Walker, S Chatterjee, J Perry, and **H Haider**
Centre for Biomedical Engineering, Institute of Orthopaedics, University College London, UK
P Campbell
Joint Replacement Institute at Orthopaedic Hospital, Los Angeles, USA
J P Paul
University of Strathclyde, Glasgow, UK

10

A New Measurement Method for Wear Scars Generated with Knee Simulators

R Konrad, C Rieker, R Schön, O Muratoglu, and **R Perinchief**

Abstract

A new measurement method, which yields significantly more information on wear behaviour than the classical visual or the widely-used gravimetric methods, has been developed for wear scars generated in knee simulators.

With this method, a co-ordinate-measuring machine is used to determine the geometry of the tibial inserts. A comparison of the initial with the final geometry of the tibial inserts facilitates the collection of information about the linear penetration and volumetric changes. Moreover, the position (anterior–posterior and medial–lateral), depth, and volume of the deformed area can be evaluated quantitatively.

This method provides new possibilities for the critical examination of wear behaviour in new designs of knee prostheses or with new polymers, such as the recently developed highly cross-linked UHMWPEs.

10.1 Introduction

After two decades of bio-tribological research focused almost exclusively on total hip prostheses, and the recent development of knee simulators, new opportunities now exist in the field of total knee prostheses. They are based primarily on the work carried out by the ISO working group ISO/TC 150.

Although there is still some controversy about the most suitable types of knee simulator (displacement-controlled, load-controlled, or with a mixed control mode), they are being used increasingly by many research groups.

In general, two methods are applied for the quantification of the deformation (creep and wear) observed after a knee simulator wear test.

10.1.1 Visual classification (1)

The visual classification provides qualitative information about the type of wear (pitting, burnishing, delamination, etc.), as well as its position and frequency on the tibial inserts. However, this method does not provide any quantitative information about the worn polyethylene volume or the penetration of the femur into the polyethylene tibial insert.

Since the worn volume of polyethylene controls the formation of cysts and osteolysis, this information is essential for the estimation of the possible long-term, *in vivo* behaviour of the knee prosthesis under test.

10.1.2 Gravimetric method (2)

The gravimetric method indicates only the total volumetric wear, but does not provide any information about the wear pattern (linear and volumetric changes induced in the articulating surfaces).

The current study presents a new method, which can provide detailed information for the quantification of the deformation induced (by both creep and wear) in tibial knee inserts after *in vitro*, knee simulator wear-testing.

10.2 Methods

The geometry of the tibial knee inserts is measured by means of a co-ordinate-measuring machine (CMM). The CMM equipment (Euro-C, Mitutoyo, Japan) has a linear measurement accuracy of better than 4 μm. The CMM measurements were carried out at the beginning of the wear test (initial geometry) and after every 500 000 or 1000 000 cycles. The measurement points followed equally spaced grids on the surface of the insert. The grid spacing was 1.0 mm in two orthogonal directions: anterior–posterior (A–P) and medial–lateral (M–L) on the tibial insert. A total of approximately 4500 measurement points were defined on the inserts. The data points were subdivided into groups of lines spanning the articulation surface in the A–P directions. These lines are designated the A–P lines. Eighty A–P lines were used for each of the inserts described in the present study.

The A–P lines measured on the tibial inserts at the beginning of the wear test were used as reference lines. The A–P lines measured during the wear test included undeformed regions at the anterior and exterior extremes and a deformed (creep and wear) region located within the central area of the insert.

The data analysis was carried out as follows:

1. The deformation scar (creep and wear) on the inserts was digitized at the end of each test interval (Fig. 10.1).
2. The position of the digitized deformation scar on the insert was superimposed electronically on the grid spacing specified by the co-ordinate measuring machine.
3. For each A–P line, the undeformed regions at the anterior and exterior extremes were compared with the original geometry after the wear test.
4. For each A–P line, a rigid-body translation and/or rotation was applied to match the undeformed regions as illustrated in Fig. 10.2.
5. The deformed area was used to reconstruct the articulating surfaces of the insert subjected to deformation through creep and wear.
6. The surfaces were triangulated and the linear as well as the volumetric differences calculated between the reference and test surfaces.

7. The deformation scar was superimposed on the initial geometry of the insert. The depth of the deformation scar was given a colour/grey code. To increase the readability of the wear scar, the linear difference was multiplied by a zoom factor. An example is shown in Fig. 10.3.

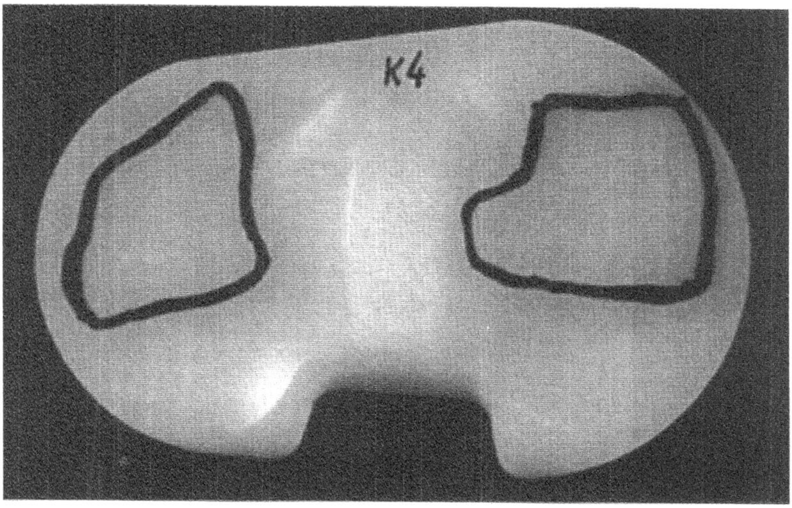

Fig. 10.1 Digitized deformation scars (creep and wear)

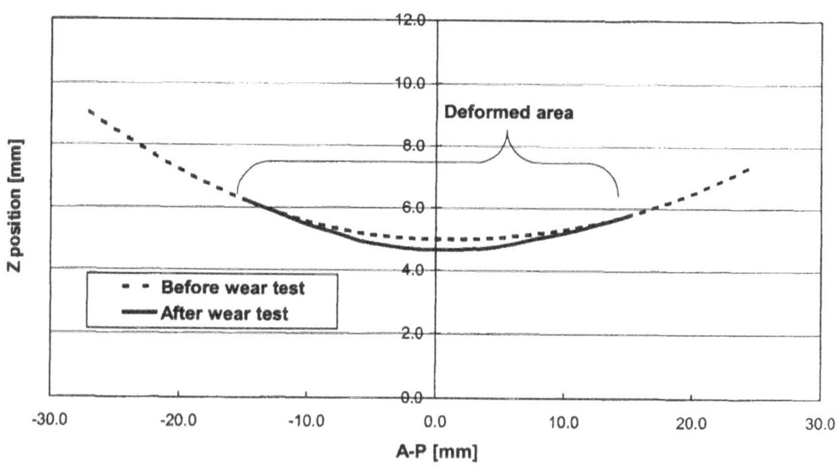

Fig. 10.2 Application of rigid-body translation and/or rotation to match the undeformed regions

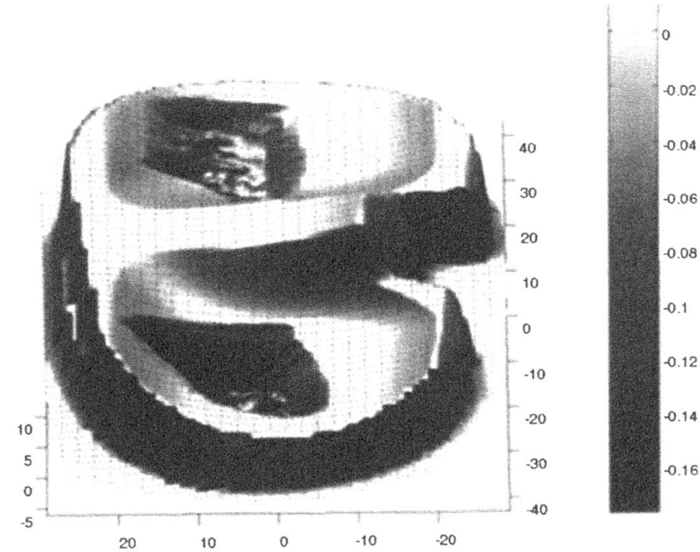

Fig. 10.3 Deformation scar

This method determined the total geometrical changes to the tibial inserts, but did not allow a differentiation between creep and wear. However, a paper published by Derbyshire *et al.* **(3)** permits creep and wear to be distinguished. Almost 100 per cent of the creep takes place during the first million cycles on the simulator. The penetration and the volume change that take place after one million cycles can therefore be regarded as wear with a negligible creep contribution. The slope of a linear regression line starting at one million cycles thus shows the penetration rate, while its offset facilitates a good estimation of the deformation due to creep.

This technique was assessed by measurements on knee prostheses (Natural-Knee II, size 3 left, Sulzer Orthopedics, Baar, Switzerland), which were tested up to 3000 000 cycles. The polyethylene inserts were manufactured in the resin 4150 and sterilized by means of gamma irradiation (2.5–4.0 MRad) in oxygen-less packaging. The lubricant used was a stabilized mixture of Ringer's solution with 33 per cent newborn calf serum (BioConcept, Allschwil, Switzerland), buffered to a pH-value of 7.2. The lubricant was also passed through a 0.2 μm filter to remove any sources of contamination and renewed every 500 000 cycles. The simulator used was a Stanmore KC knee simulator (Instron, High Wycombe, England). It is load-controlled and designed for the testing of all types of knee prostheses (hinged, fixed, or mobile bearing) with the same inputs.

10.3 Results

Figure 10.4 shows the linear penetration measured for the lateral and medial condyles. The following results were obtained:

- lateral creep 64 μm
- medial creep 42 μm
- lateral penetration rate 35 μm per million cycles
- medial penetration rate 23 μm per million cycles

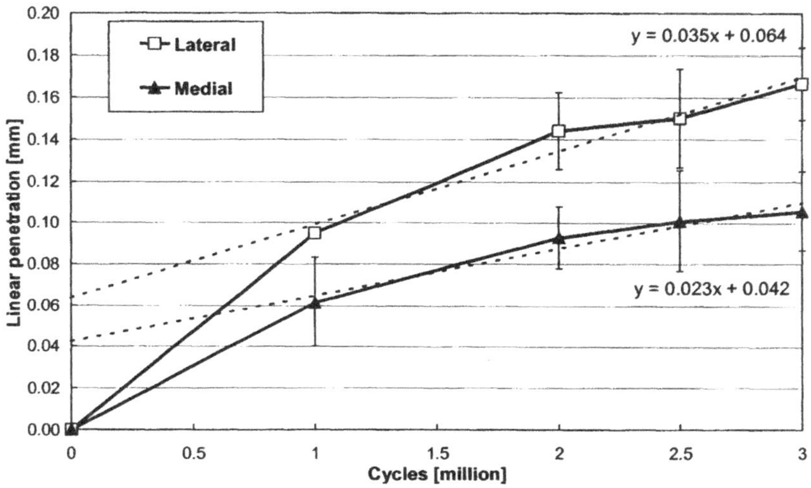

Fig. 10.4 Linear penetration for the lateral and medial condyles

Figure 10.5 indicates the global volumetric wear for the lateral and medial condyles. The following results were obtained:

- volumetric creep 10.9 mm^3
- volumetric wear rate 9.1 mm^3 per million cycles

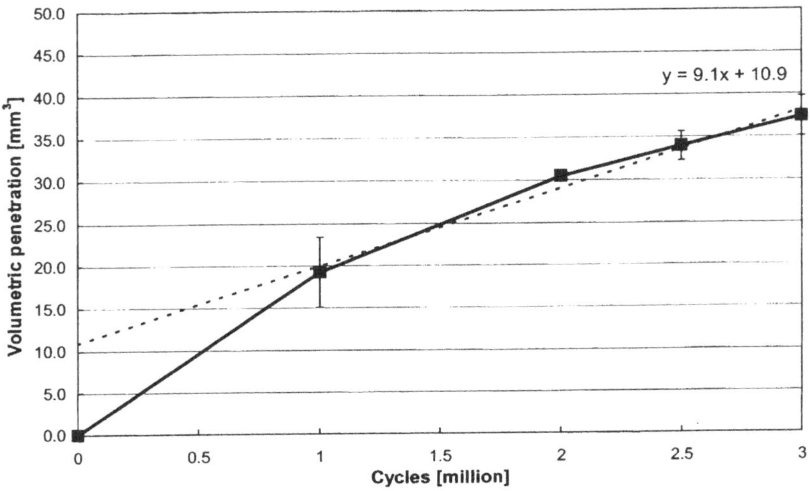

Fig. 10.5 Volumetric wear for the lateral and medial condyles

10.4 Discussion and conclusions

This newly developed method for measuring the deformation (creep and wear) in tibial inserts is a powerful tool for the assessment of the *in vitro* wear and deformation behaviour of tibial inserts. The position (anterior–posterior and medial–lateral), depth, and volume of the deformed area can be evaluated quantitatively. This method can be applied for the critical examination of the wear behaviour of new types of knee prostheses or new polymers, such as the recently developed highly cross-linked UHMWPEs.

References

(1) **Harman, M. K., Banks, S. A., Natarajan, R., Andriacchi, T. P., Hofmann, A. A.,** and **Hodge, W. A.** The spectrum of polyethylene wear in contemporary posterior cruciate ligament retaining total knee arthroplasty. *AAOS, Anaheim,* 1999, SE026.

(2) Standard guide for gravimetric wear assessment of prosthetic knee designs in simulator devices. ASTM F 1715 - 96.

(3) **Derbyshire, B., Fisher, J., Dowson, D., Hardaker, C.,** and **Brummitt, K.** Comparative study of the wear of UHMWPE with zirconia ceramic and stainless steel femoral heads in artificial hip joints, *Med Eng Phys* 1994; 16: 229–36.

R Konrad, C Rieker, and **R Schön**
Sulzer Orthopedics Limited, Winterthur, Switzerland
O Muratoglu and **R Perinchief**
Massachusetts General Hospital, Boston, Massachusetts, USA

Index

Related Titles of Interest

Title	Editor/Author	ISBN
Advances in Medical Tribology Orthopaedic Implants and Implant Materials	D Dowson	1 86058 069 6
Application of Shape Memory Alloys in Medicine	I P Lipscomb and L D M Nokes	0 85298 956 3
Guide to Wear Problems and Testing for Industry	M J Neale and M Gee	1 86058 287 7
History of Tribology	D Dowson	1 86058 070 X
IMechE Engineers' Data Book – Second Edition	C Matthews	1 86058 248 6
Introduction to the Biomechanics of Joints and Joint Replacement	D Dowson and V Wright	0 85298 384 0
Medical Applications for Shape-memory Alloys (SMA)	IMechE Seminar	1 86058 241 9
Tribology in Environmental Design	M Hadfield and C Ciantar	1 86058 266 4
Tribology – Lubrication, Friction, and Wear	I V Kragelsky and V Alisin	1 86058 288 5

For the full range of titles published by Professional Engineering Publishing contact:

Marketing Department
Professional Engineering Publishing Limited
Northgate Avenue
Bury St Edmunds
Suffolk
IP32 6BW
UK

Tel: +44 (0)1284 724384
Fax: +44 (0)1284 718692
Email: orders@pepublishing.com
Website: www.pepublishing.com

Printed and bound by CPI Group (UK) Ltd, Croydon, CR0 4YY

13/09/2026

14961030-0001